Attending

MEDICINE,
MINDFULNESS,
and HUMANITY

Ronald Epstein, M.D.

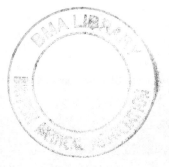

SCRIBNER

New York   London   Toronto   Sydney   New Delhi

Scribner
An Imprint of Simon & Schuster, Inc.
1230 Avenue of the Americas
New York, NY 10020

First Scribner hardcover edition January 2017

SCRIBNER and design are registered trademarks of The Gale Group, Inc., used under
license by Simon & Schuster, Inc., the publisher of this work.

For information about special discounts for bulk purchases,
please contact Simon & Schuster Special Sales at 1-866-506-1949
or business@simonandschuster.com.

The Simon & Schuster Speakers Bureau can bring authors to your live event.
For more information or to book an event, contact the Simon & Schuster Speakers
Bureau at 1-866-248-3049 or visit our website at www.simonspeakers.com.

Manufactured in the United States of America

3   5   7   9   10   8   6   4   2

Library of Congress Cataloging-in-Publication Data
Names: Epstein, Ronald, author.
Title: Attending : medicine, mindfulness, and humanity / Ronald Epstein.
Description: New York : Scribner, [2017] | Includes bibliographical
references and index.
Identifiers: LCCN 2016024695| ISBN 9781501121715 (hardcover : alk. paper) |
ISBN 9781501121722 (trade pbk. : alk. paper) | ISBN 9781501121739 (ebook)
Subjects: | MESH: Physician-Patient Relations | Mindfulness |
Physicians—psychology
Classification: LCC R690 | NLM W 62 | DDC 610.69/5—dc23 LC record available at
https://lccn.loc.gov/2016024695

ISBN 978-1-5011-2171-5
ISBN 978-1-5011-2173-9 (ebook)

Two poems of Jellaludin Rumi translated by Coleman Barks used with the
permission of Coleman Barks.

CT scan image appearing on page 18 reproduced with the author's permission.

To Deborah, Eli, and Malka,
my inspiration

Contents

Author's Note

I believe that the practice of medicine depends on a deep understanding between clinicians and patients, and that human understanding starts with understanding oneself. This book is the product of a career in medicine seeking opportunities to know myself better as a clinician and to help others do the same—ultimately to make health care more mindful, attentive, and humane. Writing this book, I've explored realms that I had not previously imagined: the cutting edge of social and cognitive neuroscience, the psychological and philosophical underpinnings of contemplative practices, and the writings of Zen masters, baseball heroes, and ecstatic poets. At each juncture, innumerable friends, colleagues, and total strangers whom I contacted out of the blue offered guidance, correctives, consolations, and camaraderie that helped me find my voice as a writer: from the heart, personal, rooted in stories.

For privacy and confidentiality, I cannot name all of my teachers. Many of them are my patients, and it would be too much to ask them to make public the most intimate moments of their lives. I have altered details of each patient's story and in some cases created a composite of two or more similar stories. Thus, any resemblance of those mentioned in this book to actual living patients and their families is coincidental and not intentional. I have taken similar precautions with the health professionals mentioned in the book, as it is difficult to know if I might unwittingly reveal something that they would rather not have made public. For convenience and readability, when referring to health professionals and patients I have used the singular pronouns *he* and *she* rather than use the more awkward *he or she* and *his or hers*. This is not to suggest any generalizations based on gender.

In medicine, the senior physician responsible for a patient's care is called the attending physician, or just "the attending." The attending's responsibility is to direct the clinical team's attention to the most important things, take charge, make the patient feel attended to, and provide attentive care. Attending means showing up, being present, listening, and accompanying patients when it matters most. Attending is also a moral imperative: by being attentive, doctors not only provide the best care, they also honor each patient's humanity.

Attending

1

Being Mindful

Even as a third-year medical student, I knew that pink was good, blue was bad.

I was assisting Mark Gunderson, a senior urologist at a university teaching hospital during my first clinical rotation in surgery. Being in the operating room was engrossing and revelatory, but I felt some trepidation about how I'd fit into the rigid hierarchy of surgical culture. Gunderson was performing a retroperitoneal lymph node dissection, painstakingly removing the lymph nodes surrounding both kidneys and the aorta. The patient, eighteen-year-old Jake Willits, had testicular cancer and the stakes were high; one false move could result in sexual dysfunction or the loss of a kidney.

After Gunderson finished operating on Jake's left kidney, we traded sides of the operating table so that he could work on the right, keeping the left kidney within his peripheral vision. I had a straight-on view of the left kidney. After a few minutes, I noticed that the kidney was turning blue. Gunderson didn't seem to have noticed.

I agonized about what to do. As a lowly medical student, I knew it wasn't my place to offer an opinion to a senior surgeon, but I felt compelled to speak up: "I'm not sure you've got a good view, but the left kidney is looking bluish to me." I spoke loudly enough to be heard, but tentatively enough so as not to appear arrogant. No response. Gunderson asked the scrub nurse for a scalpel. His gaze didn't move. I became increasingly anxious and broke into a sweat.

After a few more minutes, the kidney had turned an ominous dusky purple. I quietly mentioned this to the scrub nurse at my side, who talked to the resident, who then talked to the surgeon.

Gunderson looked and didn't like what he saw. The left kidney had become twisted, blocking blood flow through the renal artery. He tried to untwist the kidney, first one way, then the other. No success. The room became tense and quiet. Now Gunderson was sweating too, knowing that with each passing minute a few more kidney cells would die. After what seemed like an eternity but was probably only a few minutes, Gunderson called in a vascular surgeon to do an urgent repair of the renal artery. Apparently, when the kidney twisted, the intima—the inner lining of the renal artery—had been torn, blocking blood flow. The vascular surgeon had to clamp the artery, make a longitudinal slice, open up the injured area, and excise the torn fragment—delicately, while leaving the outer layers of the artery intact—then sew up the artery. This mishap extended the operation by more than an hour, and while the operation was successful, blood tests just afterward showed that Jake's kidney function was not quite normal. While the surgery likely cured Jake of his cancer, no one knew when—or if—his kidney would fully recover. The next morning, on rounds, Gunderson informed Jake and his parents that an "unavoidable" complication had occurred.[1]

Today when I tell this story to an audience of doctors, I always see nods of understanding. I know that this situation does not mean that Gunderson is a "bad doctor"; so do they. Surgery is difficult and intense, and errors are easy to make. Even the most experienced clinicians—surgeons and otherwise—can suffer lapses of attention and ignore that which in retrospect seems obvious.[2]

The kidney getting twisted might have been unavoidable. But Gunderson's failure to notice and act was not. He was focused, for sure. But his inattention to that which was in plain sight—even after it was pointed out to him—was stunning, especially given that he was an accomplished surgeon at a major teaching hospital. Certainly, the light reflected by the blue kidney was picked up by his retina, and no doubt his ears could detect what I had said. Nevertheless, something happened in that crucial moment to prevent that visual and auditory data from being fully transmitted to his conscious awareness. In essence, Gunderson hadn't engaged his whole mind.

This event had a powerful impact on me. I realized how easily I could put my patients' lives at risk in a similar way. I was distraught. I lost sleep wondering if I had done something wrong; perhaps, I thought, if I had spoken up more assertively, Jake wouldn't have suffered as much damage to his kidney. And I felt uncomfortable allowing the family to believe that the surgeon was blameless.

I made an appointment to speak with the chief of surgery the next week. I asked if I could talk confidentially. He was a good listener and assured me that I had done the right thing by talking to him and that the mishap was in no way my fault. He was visibly concerned and assured me that he would talk with the surgeon and check in with Jake and his family. We discharged Jake a few days later, in good spirits.

I never saw Gunderson again, and unfortunately I could never know what he truly believed. While I was upset that an error had occurred, it wasn't a surprise to me that even the most expert surgeons could be fallible. The most important lessons, though, were that mindless inattention could result in disaster and that competence is fragile and takes mindful vigilance to maintain. This experience planted the seed of an idea in me—that I'd need not only skill and expertise, but something else to be the doctor I wanted to be, something no one had spent much time teaching me in medical school: the ability to be self-aware, attentive, and present, especially when the stakes were high. I'd need to be a guardian of my patients' health and *also* of my own "inner operating system" in each moment.[3] Awareness of my own mind might be one of the most important tools I could have in addressing patients' needs.

I thought of this event again later that month, while working with Ashwin Mehta, a vascular surgeon at the same hospital. When I arrived at the operating room, Mehta had already made a large incision in Lena Hagopian's abdomen. Mehta was moving quickly, tying and cutting sutures faster than I could count. I couldn't help but notice his focus and intensity, his large hands moving rapidly and decisively as he got ready to repair a cholesterol-clogged aorta to open up blood flow to the patient's oxygen-starved legs. Soft rock music played in the background as he worked and bantered with the operating room staff. Then, suddenly, the bantering stopped. The operating room grew quiet, a silence different from Gunderson's. The time had come to sew a large blood vessel back together, a procedure that required delicacy and precision. But, the anastomosis—the connection between the two parts of the blood vessel—was leaking. Unlike Gunderson, Mehta noticed that something was awry before anyone else did. By the time *we* realized it, Mehta had already shifted seamlessly from autopilot to more deliberately choreographed action—first tango, then ballet, then a few minutes later back to tango—all without missing a beat. No panic, only calm focus, surgical mindfulness in action. His shifting of gears was so smooth that I wondered if he was even aware of it.[4]

Only decades later did I understand. A surgeon colleague, Carol-Anne Moulton, made the connection for me. She was researching what made great surgeons great and had observed dozens of surgeons performing complex operations. She had documented in detail how during difficult moments masterful surgeons would shift gears. Those who "slowed down when they should" when encountering speed bumps were the true masters; those who kept going full speed ahead tended to make errors.[5] Mehta had slowed down when he should.

Yet when Moulton interviewed surgeons about these slowing down moments, many of the masters didn't realize that they had shifted gears until it was pointed out to them, and only upon reflection could they put into words exactly what triggered them to make the shift. Mehta was not any more technically skilled or knowledgeable than Gunderson; that's not what made him a master. His expertise resided in his exquisite moment-to-moment awareness: he was able to be present and to bring what was needed to each moment. While operating on Mrs. Hagopian, he could also monitor his own inner operating system so that he would realize when he might need to slow down or get help. He accepted and anticipated the possibility that something could go wrong. Whether he thought about it this way or not, Mehta was being mindful.

I discovered that mindfulness is also essential outside the operating room. Later in my third year, I worked with a senior psychiatrist, Dr. Peter Reich. Reich eventually became a mentor—from the first time I met him, I felt drawn to him by his thoughtfulness, insight, and curiosity about the human condition. At that time, he was responsible for the care of medically ill patients in the hospital who also presented mental health problems. Halfway through the one-month rotation, he and I were called to the neurology unit to see Douglas McCallum, a man in his thirties who had sustained a head injury in a motorcycle accident. Doug was not cooperating with the specialists handling his rehabilitation program; he was moody and irritable and had angry outbursts that frightened the staff. Part of his brain was damaged, the part that had made him the Doug that he and others had known. You could see Doug trying to make sense of his situation, yet his thoughts would leap from one topic to the next and he was unable to retrieve what he had just been saying. His thinking was fragmented. He was frightened because he knew that something was very wrong. He had become a stranger to himself.

The medical team wanted Dr. Reich to help manage Doug's erratic behavior. Reich had a long list of patients to see; given that this one had apparently irreversible brain damage, I expected Reich to assign a diagnosis quickly and prescribe medications to control Doug's behavior—something I had witnessed other psychiatrists doing under similar circumstances. To my surprise, Reich did something radical: he temporarily set aside the imperative to diagnose and treat so that he could get to know Doug as a person. He asked, "What does that feel like?" and "Help me understand." Reich nodded and smiled kindly, indicating that he was not in a rush and was fully engaged. He sought to discover what *was* working in Doug's mind, as well as what wasn't.

While surgeons' tools are scalpels and forceps, Reich's tools were words and gestures. His interview with Doug would flow smoothly for a while, with Doug appearing almost coherent, remembering details and the order in which things occurred. Then Doug would freeze, unable to complete a thought. The circuits were jammed. These uncomfortable pauses reminded us how seriously his mind had gone awry.

Reich was mindful in the same ways as Mehta—he was attending and present—but I could see that there was more to mindfulness than attention and presence. Reich was curious about Doug's experience.[6] He set aside preconceptions so he could see Doug in a new way. As impressed as I was by Reich's ability to help Doug construct a coherent narrative from a set of disorganized thoughts, I also noticed that Reich was gently persistent during those awkward moments. When Doug abruptly transitioned from one story to another with no logical connector—talking about riding his motorcycle the previous week and then about a camping trip with his brother twenty years prior—Reich encouraged him, saying, "What happened next?" If Doug's reply still didn't make sense, Reich would add, "Are you feeling sometimes that things aren't making sense?" That helped Doug achieve enough clarity to say, "Yep, my thoughts just come and go."

Reich was shifting back and forth between an expert's perspective—making a diagnosis—and a "beginner's mind," stepping into Doug's chaos rather than merely diagnosing it. Reich's openness allowed him to achieve an understanding of the patient as a person without imposing interpretations or judgments. How easy it would have been to reduce Doug to a category, a diagnosis, a problem to be solved. As Doug's attending physician, Reich understood that Doug needed to feel understood, and the more Doug felt understood, the less he'd need to express his distress through disruptive behavior. Reich's resolve to share his patient's experience, rather than ignoring it, distracting himself, or turning away, was courageous and compassionate. He responded to Doug's need—as a suffering human being—to feel understood and cared for, and in that way reaffirmed Doug's humanity.

TURNING INWARD

Mehta and Reich demonstrated to me what was possible. Their habits of mind and presence seemed instinctive. I'm not even sure Mehta and Reich could fully explain what made them mindful during those critical moments. I saw how awareness, flexibility, and attention are crucial for all clinicians, regardless of specialty or profession.

The question was how to get there. Because of the paucity of attention to self-awareness during medical education, I had to rely on other experiences. In my teens, I studied piano, then harpsichord, hoping to be a performing musician—self-awareness of my breathing, tension, heartbeat, and emotions made the difference between a performance that was technically adept and one that sparkled. When I was sixteen, I learned how to meditate. I spent an evening with a friend's older brother who was a serious student of Zen Buddhism; he taught me how. In my first semester at college, I took a course called Emptiness.[7] In Buddhist philosophy, the concept of emptiness is fundamental; it means that much of what we believe about the world—and about ourselves—is merely an "empty" construct of our own mind and limits us unnecessarily. When you see the world only as perilous, you're correct, but you're only seeing half of the picture. The world is also safe and nurturing. To see it either way alone is incomplete—it is both. When you see yourself only as infallible, you are more likely to miss a blue kidney. When you see yourself only as fallible, you can feel paralyzed. Jon Kabat-Zinn, who popularized mindfulness training in the West, said that being unaware of the labels we place on ourselves is like being in a "straightjacket of unconsciousness."[8] You have no place to move, no place to grow. Emptiness, on the other hand, is being able to see yourself as fallible and infallible at the same time.[9] You are self-assured and confident, but equally aware that you could make an error at any moment. This vision frees you to be whom you need to be—and to do what you need to do—in each moment. Yet freedom takes work—the hard work of being still and cultivating an inner life.

I got a glimpse of that freedom and I wanted more. I left college to spend a few months at the San Francisco Zen Center. Doing sitting meditation for several hours every day was both easy and difficult. I learned that when I had strong feelings—restlessness, impatience, avoidance, self-criticism, loneliness, or fear—I could just *be with* those feelings without having to alter them in any way. I felt centered and resilient, with a sense of dynamic stability. I learned that meditation is not about bliss. Meditation is about a sense of presence, balance, and connection with what is most fundamentally important in your life. It is not about leading a cloistered life; in fact, my time at the Zen Center led me to engage more fully with the world.

Eventually I wanted to translate what I had learned about the inner life so that I could make a difference in the world, and I reconnected with a childhood desire to be a doctor. Yet I was ill prepared for the culture of medical school. I had spent much of my youth in seminars, music studios, and Zen meditation halls. Med school was an environment of extremes. Altogether, I saw too much harshness, mindlessness, and inhumanity. Medical school was dominated by facts, pathways, and mechanisms; residency was about learning to diagnose, treat, and do procedures, framed by a pit-of-the-stomach dread that you might kill someone by missing something or not knowing enough. Given the life-and-death stakes, I found it jarring that, with few exceptions, medical training did not emphasize deep listening—to oneself or to others. While extolling the virtues of reflection and compassion, medical training largely ignores the development of these capacities—and an inner life in general. I felt disappointed and alone and didn't see a path forward.

Then, Reich sent me a groundbreaking article by George Engel about a "biopsychosocial" approach to care.[10] Engel was a prominent internist and psychoanalyst who practiced and taught at the University of Rochester. I wrote to him, and eventually he became a mentor. Engel showed, through exploring patients' illness experience, how patients' psychological makeup and social relationships were as important to illness and health as the biological, genetic, and molecular aspects of disease. His vision was humanistic; using dazzling illustrations, Engel demonstrated that what the patient reported about his illness and how it affected him was as important as any lab test or X-ray. Engel emphasized that physicians are human too—that their emotional responses to uncertainty, tragedy, grief, and loss would affect the care they provide.[11] This resonated with me. Doctoring was a relationship between two people, each of whom had an inner life. I moved to Rochester and worked with Engel and several of his protégés. Engel was fascinated with human experience, but, in my view, was too much of the cold scientist to offer a method for knowing one's inner life more intimately. Several of his protégés filled that role for me. Trained by Engel, they took his work one step further and offered opportunities for reflection, self-awareness, and mindfulness (so-called Balint groups,[12] family-of-origin groups,[13] personal awareness groups,[14] and clinical supervision[15]) that were available in few other settings at the time.

Over time I became more comfortable with my level of knowledge and skill as a clinician, yet I still knew that each day, with each patient, sometimes I was the physician I aspired to be and other times I fell short. Falling short had little to do with knowledge and technique, but rather it had to do with my state of mind, what I noticed and attended to. Sometimes I practiced with clarity and compassion, and other times impatience, distraction, unexamined emotions, and defensiveness got in the way.

Lacking a guidebook, I had to look inside myself. Then I'd match up my states of mind with what I had been learning about the sciences of mind—psychology, philosophy, education, and neuroscience. Wading through a profusion of educational and psychological jargon,[16] I came to three conclusions—good doctors need to be self-aware to practice at their best; self-awareness needs to be in the moment, not just Monday-morning quarterbacking; and no one had a road map.[17]

Ten years after I finished my residency, the connections between my prior training in meditation and music and my medical practice finally crystallized. My dean tasked me with developing a new method for assessing the competence of students that would reflect the biopsychosocial values that Rochester had become known for—no small undertaking. I could find few guideposts, not even a coherent definition of professional competence.[18] I wanted to capture the habits of master clinicians, those to whom doctors might refer a friend or relative, as opposed to those who were merely competent—those who merely aced the test.[19] I started writing about "mindful practice"; I drafted a personal manifesto about excellence in clinical practice and proposed that mindful self-awareness, self-monitoring, and self-regulation were at the root of good judgment, compassion, and attentive care. I had not seen a similar vision articulated before, and I had no idea how it would be received.

The manuscript went back and forth to the *Journal of the American Medical Association* seven times, and each time Charlene Breedlove, my insightful and patient editor, asked me to clarify, hone, and condense before "Mindful Practice" finally went to press in 1999.[20] The article struck a chord. I discovered that I was not alone. I received hundreds of letters and e-mails from other physicians. These practitioners, many of whom had found some form of contemplative practice on their own, felt isolated and in need of a community that would support their efforts to become more mindful, resilient, self-aware, and effective. I was deeply gratified, yet the next steps—to see if mindfulness makes a difference in patient care and how to help clinicians be more mindful—were daunting.

IN THE CLINIC

My colleague Dr. Mary Catherine Beach, at Johns Hopkins, helped to provide an answer. She studied interactions between patients and doctors in AIDS clinics around the United States.[21] People with HIV/AIDS often feel stigmatized and misunderstood, and not surprisingly, many are distrustful of the health care system. Beach and her team audio-recorded visits between doctors and patients and surveyed them afterward, including assessments of mindfulness. Physicians who were more mindful did better at developing rapport, following up on patients' concerns, and addressing psychosocial issues; their patients felt better understood, more connected, and emotionally supported. Mindful physicians won their patients' trust, no trivial matter. A patient's trust in her physician is the best predictor of whether she will take her medications, a crucial factor if you're HIV infected. Missing even a few doses could allow the virus to replicate and become drug resistant. Connection, understanding, and trust are essential.

Still, Beach's study did not answer whether practicing physicians could be *trained* to be more mindful and, if so, whether they would provide better care. For years it had been known that mindfulness training could help patients with a variety of mental and physical disorders. Yet the idea of mindfulness for physicians to enhance their *own* work was new. I found like-minded colleagues—Mick Krasner, Tim Quill, Tony Suchman, Howard Beckman, and others at the University of Rochester—and together we designed a year-long program in mindful practice for experienced primary care physicians.[22] The sessions included different kinds of meditation practice and exercises to promote mindful communication, emphasizing how to bring mindfulness into clinicians' everyday work to help them be attentive and aware. Each session touched on a particular issue—responding to errors, witnessing suffering, facing uncertainty, grieving the loss of a patient, developing compassion, feeling attracted to patients, and others. We also addressed clinician burnout directly, knowing that burned-out physicians provide lower-quality care and are more likely to quit practice altogether. We drew a simple model of what we were trying to do—the technical quality of care, the qualities of caring, and clinicians' resilience and well-being—showing how these three domains were linked and how practicing mindfully could affect all three. We started out with a group of seventy physicians, nearly all of whom scored high on a burnout questionnaire. We didn't know if they'd have the energy and commitment to finish the program or if it would show any positive effects at all.

The results far exceeded our expectations.[23] Physicians' well-being improved and their burnout decreased. They became more empathic and oriented toward their patients' psychosocial needs. We were astonished that they scored higher on conscientiousness and emotional stability, key features of personality that aren't sup-

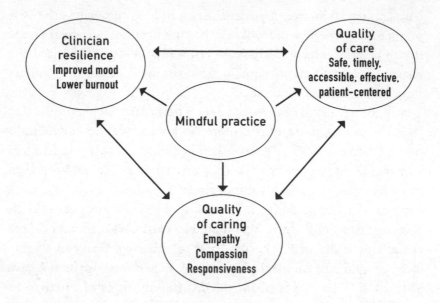

posed to change in people in their forties and fifties (more about this in chapter 10).[24] They became more attentive and focused, less likely to be derailed by crises, and better able to rely on their inner resources to remain resilient. We interviewed some of the doctors a year later. They continued to affirm that cultivating a practice of mindfulness, creating a community of supportive colleagues, and giving themselves permission to focus on their own growth made them better physicians. They reconnected with the reasons they went into medicine in the first place: to provide effective and humanistic care, and to have meaningful relationships with their patients.[25] They set limits and had a more balanced work life.

A MINDFUL VISION

Medicine is in crisis. Physicians and patients are disillusioned, frustrated by the fragmentation of the health care system. Patients cannot help but notice that I spend more and more time looking at computer screens and less time face-to-face.[26] They experience the consequences of the commodification of medicine that has forced clinicians' focus from the healing of patients to the mechanics of health care—productivity pressures, insurance regulations, actuarial tasks, and demoralizing metrics that measure what can be counted and not what really counts, sometimes ironically in the name of evidence-based and patient-centered care.[27]

I have seen that it is possible to do better, and that is the reason I'm writing this book. Amid this crisis in health care, some physicians are making choices to reacquaint themselves with the heart of medical practice. By looking inward, they are expanding their capacity to provide high-quality care. They are seeing how they, as doctors, have the power to transform and humanize the practice of medicine and how patients can be better consumers of health care, build stronger relationships with their physicians, and identify those who can provide the care they need.

Mindful practice in medicine is more than meditation and personal growth.[28] Being mindful is when I know to stop briefly, look a patient in the eye, and ask, "Have I got it all, or is there more?"—and a patient, whose previously well-controlled diabetes is now uncontrolled, then tells me he hasn't been taking care of himself since his wife died six months ago. It's when I inject an inflamed shoulder joint—with focused attention, visualizing the bones, tendons, and muscles—and the needle slides in easily and painlessly. I'm being mindful when I notice that a patient doesn't look quite right, not her usual self, and then I notice the fatigued expression and the faint rash that are clues to her new diagnosis of lupus. Attending to each patient means that I remember that, although the last patient I saw has only days to live, the next patient—with a stubbed toe—needs the same focused attention.

Medicine and *meditation*, etymologically, come from the same root: to consider, advise, reflect, to take appropriate measures. But while I can try to describe what being mindful is like, words carry just so far; ultimately, mindfulness is an experience—something that we have all encountered at some moment. Perhaps, as you are reading, you might periodically stop for a moment and become aware of your own body and your thoughts, emotions, and expectations; be aware of how present, curious, engaged, and attentive you are feeling. Over time, you will know yourself better. For starters, let this be an invitation to know the lens through which you view the world.

2

Attending

You can observe a lot by just watching.
— Yogi Berra[1]

Emil Laszlo, a sixty-six-year-old Hungarian-American engineer, had been a patient of mine for several years. An avid tennis player, he had had few medical problems other than a bout of rotator-cuff tendinitis of his right shoulder two years prior. Upon my return from a trip, I was surprised to discover an urgent voice mail from his wife. Emil was in the hospital. I called her back and she explained that the doctors suspected that he had cancer. But she was confused because they had seen three different clinicians in my absence, and after each visit to our clinic they had left with the idea that his right shoulder pain was nothing more than a recurrent rotator-cuff problem.

I investigated his chart for clues. On his first visit he saw one of my practice partners. The chart noted that Emil had pain in his right shoulder and it felt as if "there was a swelling there." The physical exam confirmed tenderness and pain on motion, but there was no description of the "swelling." Unlike two years before, though, he did not have some of the typical signs of rotator-cuff tendinitis—such as decreased range of motion or muscle weakness. It wasn't unreasonable to think that this might be a recurrence of his tendinitis; weakness and restriction of motion might not be present early in the clinical course. He was sent home with typical advice for rotator-cuff injuries: a prescription for a nonsteroidal anti-inflammatory medication and physical-therapy exercises. Yet the chart also mentioned that Emil felt feverish and had had a few night sweats. Perhaps because it was flu season, I presume, his doctors had a convenient explanation.

At Emil's second visit to our office, the physician noted a "prominence" near the shoulder. Again, full range of motion. She attributed the "history of night sweats" to a "viral syndrome." Emil also came with several additional concerns: mild prostate-related symptoms, fatigue, and a low vitamin D level. She encouraged him to continue with physical therapy and anti-inflammatory medications, and I can only assume that she thought that the prominence was related to his rotator-cuff problem. Notably, she did not call it a "lump" or a "mass" or anything that might connote something more serious.

On the third visit, he reported worsening fatigue, more than you would expect from the flu. His pain was worsening despite medications and exercise. Yet, the chart still didn't mention a mass. The nurse-practitioner homed in on his disabling fatigue and ordered some blood tests. The results showed an extremely low white blood count. She called Emil at home and sent him to the emergency room. Only then, after the blood test suggested something serious might be going on, was the ten-centimeter tumor extending from his armpit to his shoulder finally "seen." In hindsight it all made sense—pain, a mass, and fatigue are typical for lymphoma—but all three clinicians were stunned by the news and were at a loss to explain how they could have missed something so obvious.[2]

Every day, clinicians fail to attend to something that seems obvious in hindsight. Emil's situation got me wondering why. Clinical care is fast paced. Amid a deluge of patients with potentially preventable acute problems, poorly controlled chronic diseases, and intractable mental health issues, and whose uncooperative insurance companies won't pay for medicines they need, Emil arrives. To his physician's relief, Emil seems to have a problem that is straightforward and easy to solve. I wondered if his clinicians' (mis)diagnoses had to do with misperception (Did they not even look or did they look and not really see the tumor?), misinterpretation (Did they see it yet misjudge its significance?), misprioritization (Because it didn't "make sense" was it relegated to secondary status?), or closed-mindedness (Having arrived at one explanation, did the clinician lose interest in seeking out alternative explanations?). All of these factors can contribute to what psychologists call *inattentional blindness*.

We all experience inattentional blindness in everyday life. Often it is of little consequence; you find your keys in the place where you just looked. Other times it is more serious. A friend of mine had a rear-end collision on a sunny fall morning; he was talking on his hands-free mobile phone and didn't see the car right in front of him. Or take this well-known example: In a video that has gone viral, players dressed in black outfits and white outfits toss a basketball, and the viewer is instructed to count the number of passes between the players in white. The majority of viewers are oblivious of someone in a black gorilla suit moonwalking across the set—until it is pointed out to them.[3] It had been filtered out. Filtering is a neurologic necessity to keep us from being overwhelmed by all the stimuli from the environment; below our awareness, our brains make choices, usually the right ones, but sometimes the wrong ones—especially when the stimulus is unexpected.

Even those who are exquisitely trained to look for visual details miss the unexpected. In one study, a researcher asked radiologists to view a chest CT scan on a computer screen. A small gorilla figure was strategically placed in one of the images. More than three-quarters of the radiologists didn't notice the gorilla. Unbeknownst to the radiologists, the computer had sophisticated visual-tracking technology that confirmed that their eyes had looked directly at it.[4] Their inattentional blindness had little to do with knowledge and years of experience.

Inattentional deafness works the same way: it's an auditory glitch in which we don't hear things that are clearly said to us. More than once I've had a worried parent bring a child to my office for a hearing test, hoping for an explanation for why the child doesn't respond when spoken to, only to find that the hearing is perfect.

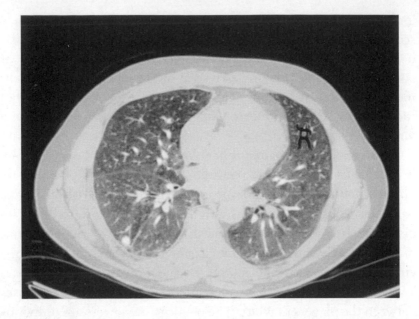

(This happens with married couples too!) As a clinician, I can so easily not hear the unexpected and the unwanted. Like inattentional blindness, it can be benign or life-threatening; in the operating room, it could be fatal.[5]

How can this happen? Research shows how focusing intensely on a visual task—in the operating room or looking at a computer screen—interferes with our ability to listen.[6] The reverse is likely true too; that is why talking on cell phones while driving—even with hands-free devices—leads to accidents. We can't pay attention to everything all the time. Like computers, our brains have a limited capacity for *working memory*—that which we can hold in our awareness at any given moment—and our brains are constantly making choices. More accurately, we prioritize that which is personally meaningful and ignore sensory input that we consider to be of low value—information that is inconsistent with our expectations or information that comes from a presumably unreliable source (such as a third-year medical student). The problem is that these "choices" are usually below our levels of awareness, and thus we don't routinely assess the rational or irrational factors that go into making them.

NOT SEEING, NOT KNOWING

The great physician-teacher William Osler once said, "We miss more by not seeing than by not knowing." It may sound trivial, but simply paying attention is one of the most difficult tasks for clinicians. It's no secret that much of what physicians do is routine. Reading an electrocardiogram or prescribing medications for hypothyroidism or heart failure is often done by protocol, and to save working memory, our brains make most of those tasks automatic, or nearly so. We use what psychologist Daniel Kahneman calls Type 1 processing, or fast thinking.[7] Anyone, even without a medical background, could easily learn the symptoms and treatments for urinary tract infections and get it right about 80 percent of the time. But in 20 percent of the situations, something atypical appears and requires that doctors switch out of autopilot and apply a more conscious, focused attention, what Kahneman calls Type 2 or slow thinking. Medical training is long and arduous largely to help doctors deal with the 20 percent, the unexpected and complex situations that require more than just knowledge, technical skills, and years of experience.[8] Yet doctors aren't trained to notice and make the switch from automatic thinking to a slower—more deliberative—mode. It's easy not to notice the unexpected, especially once we've committed ourselves to a provisional idea about what might be going on.

For twenty-five years I've studied communication in health care settings. As a communications researcher, I notice how physicians systematically pay attention to some kinds of information more than others. It is particularly alarming how often physicians are oblivious to patients' emotional distress, despite their providing clues that they are afraid, distrustful, confused, or depressed. Patients will say, "I'm tired," "Just shoot me," "My sister's cancer is progressing," and get little acknowledgment.[9] In one study of thoracic surgeons seeing patients with lung cancer, over 90 percent of the emotional content of conversations went unacknowledged.[10] Admittedly, some physicians intentionally ignore emotional content, feeling that is not their job (I disagree).[11] Yet, when reviewing audio-recordings of their consultations, physicians are often surprised at how many of those concerns went unheard.

A few years ago, I set out to understand how this kind of inattention happens in primary care. I trained actors to pose as patients with chest pain who made appointments to see primary care physicians in the Rochester area. The doctors had previously consented to participate in the research, but had no idea when the actors would come and what symptoms they might present. The roles were constructed so that the actors were likely to escape detection. Generally it worked. The vast majority of the time physicians thought that they were real patients. In an intentional effort to simulate the ambiguities of primary care practice, the actors portrayed chest pain that was not typical of heart disease, heartburn (gastroesophageal reflux, or GERD), or musculoskeletal pain; sometimes it would be worse with movement or after eating or at night, with no pattern to the symptoms. We also trained the actors to ask the doctors a key question: "Could this be something serious?"

We were intentionally trying to increase physicians' cognitive load, to force them to choose among competing explanations for the patient's symptoms. One doctor said to the patient, "Maybe this is heartburn, let's get an EKG." While an EKG might provide useful information about the heart, it would certainly not help diagnose heartburn. The physicians were befuddled.

Furthermore, when patients asked the "something serious" question, few received any empathy or even acknowledgment of their worry.[12] Rather, physicians tended to ask further questions about physical symptoms, provide bland reassurance or more medical information, or change the topic. If these had been real patients, their fears might have been compounded, or they might have felt sheepish that they had brought up a trivial concern. This might affect their future decisions about when to seek health care and from whom.

I met with a focus group of physicians after the study. None said that they thought their patient's emotional distress was trivial. Rather, they said that they just didn't register the emotional content, that diagnosis and medications were more on their radar.

Cognitive load drove them to distraction. Clearly, talking about serious illness is difficult for both clinicians and patients, and some physicians consciously avoid such discussions. But if these physicians had a moment-to-moment awareness of their own attentional choices, most would have prefaced their response with "I can see how concerned you are about this."

There is some good news, though. Given the opportunity, physicians can be keen detectors of their own blind spots—they can raise that which is just below the level of awareness into consciousness. In a study from the 1990s, I asked physicians to watch video-recordings of their consultations with their patients who were at high risk for AIDS.[13] These patients were often terrified; at that time the treatments for AIDS were not effective. Patients not only feared the disease; they also feared stigmatization. When patients expressed distress, physicians often missed it.

When the doctors reviewed their video-recordings, they were shocked—just as people watching the basketball video a second time couldn't believe that they missed the gorilla. One doctor was mortified when he viewed himself asking questions about intimate sexual behavior (a good thing) as he was performing a testicular exam (not exactly the way to make a young male patient feel less vulnerable). While missing the gorilla in an online video generates amusement and wonder, missing emotions or causing humiliation in the examining room has real and important consequences—the physician may have missed an opportunity to detect and treat the HIV infection before it progressed to AIDS. Patients who feel unheard are less likely to disclose important information and less likely to follow their doctors' recommendations.[14]

I CAN'T HEAR YOU WHILE I'M LISTENING

You might think that if you were in a quiet, controlled setting, such as an exam room, it would be relatively effortless to pay attention. While lack of distraction helps, it's not enough. In a brilliant article from the 1980s, primary care internist Richard Baron wrote about a time when he was listening to a patient's heart with a stethoscope. The patient started talking (uncanny how often they do), and Baron said, "Quiet . . . I can't hear you while I'm listening."[15] While technically true that it is hard to hear speech through a stethoscope and virtually impossible to hear subtle breath sounds and heart murmurs when a patient is talking, it points to the realities of medical practice: that our moment-to-moment choices reside just below our level of conscious awareness, somewhat like our awareness of what's in our peripheral vision.[16] Stimuli compete for clinicians' attention in a time-pressured, psychologically demanding, and unforgiving environment. Clinicians need the ability to focus their attention on the task at hand, while also having access to their subsidiary awareness—perceptions that are just below the surface of awareness.

Learning how attention works is important to both doctors and patients. I know, for example, that long-winded rambles and repetitive descriptions of symptoms by patients tire me, yet buried in their ramblings might be clues to something serious. With practice, I might be able to avert missing something important by increasing my awareness of my attentional habits and blind spots and switch more adeptly between autopilot and focused attention; like a "mental muscle," the capacity for attention can be grown and developed.

Patients can help too. As a patient, when you don't get the information or understanding that you need, you can say, "I just want to make sure I've been clear about ____." Or "I'm particularly worried about ____." Or "I'm not sure I understand what that means." This can help you and your doctor focus on what's most important. Just as doctors need practice to communicate effectively, patients also need practice in assertive communication. It pays off in two ways: you're more likely to reorient your physician's attention toward your needs and you are more likely to get an answer that makes sense. Knowing about inattentional deafness means that you can appreciate that a lack of response from a physician may mean that you've simply not been heard, and not that your concern is unimportant (especially when your doctor has the stethoscope in her ears or is typing on a computer). Fortunately, in conversation, with more flexible parsing of our attention, we can recalibrate and go back to clarify something that has been missed or misunderstood.

The fast pace of clinical practice—accelerated by electronic records—requires juggling multiple tasks seemingly simultaneously. Although commonly thought of as multitasking, multitasking is a misnomer—we actually alternate among tasks. Each time we switch tasks we need time to recover and, during the recovery period, we are less effective. Psychologists call this interruption recovery failure, which sounds a bit like those computer error messages we all dread. We increasingly feel as if we are victims of distractions rather than in control of them.[17]

In addition to information that comes from the outside world, we are constantly processing information that comes from the "sixth sense"—the mind itself. While focusing on a task (for a physician it might be examining a patient's abdomen or suturing a wound), we all have spontaneously arising thoughts, emotions, and visceral sensations that may or may not relate directly to the situation at hand. If you have any doubt about the constant flow of these mental events, take a couple of minutes, close your eyes, and simply watch the flow of sensations, feelings, thoughts, and emotions, without trying to alter them in any way. We doubt ourselves, remind ourselves about other tasks, feel anxious or sad, and notice grumblings in our stomach or tension in our shoulders.

The brain strives for efficiency. Under high cognitive load—when assaulted with difficult problems, too much information, and emotional stress—the brain tends to simplify. It privileges familiar and expected information and relatively ignores that which is novel, unpleasant, or unexpected.[18] In clinical practice, I find that I tend to pay closer attention to the first thing—or the last thing—that the patient says. When Emil Laszlo mentioned his vitamin D level and prostate symptoms in addition to his shoulder pain, he was unknowingly adding to his physician's cognitive load just by virtue of presenting more concerns. In medicine, the imperative to simplify often leads to premature closure—after reaching a certain information threshold, the brain admits no more information, comes to a conclusion, and treats that conclusion as fact. At that point, we tend to consider only that which confirms our initial impression (shoulder pain and a history of tendinitis), and to ignore the rest (fever, sweats, and a lump). Overconfidence and hurry make matters worse. While inattention is the starting point for many failures of clinical reasoning and empathy, the lack of awareness can undermine effective and humanistic care in many other ways.

TOP-DOWN

During the surgery described at the beginning of this book, Dr. Gunderson, the resident, and the nurse were all focused on the right kidney, and with good reason. They wanted to bring their visual awareness, motor skills, and judgment to a delicate task. They knew that with one false move, things could go sour. Their minds were processing vast quantities and varieties of complex sensory information. They needed to anticipate the likely challenges and come up with a game plan. The surgeon might have had an inner dialogue: "Need to be careful not to injure the ureter, so I'll focus exclusively on that part of the anatomy for now."

Goal-directed attention is also known as top-down attention, or orienting attention. It is about anticipating something that is known and expected with heightened vigilance. Although we like to think that we're in control of our minds, most of our thought process occurs outside our everyday awareness.[19] While top-down attention can go awry, as we've seen, it usually serves us well. To take an everyday example, on my short commute to work there is a stop sign at the corner of Hemingway Drive and Elmwood Avenue. As I approach Elmwood, my mind is primed to see that stop sign and to respond accordingly—even though I'm not aware of thinking about it. In clinical practice, when I see a child with a fever, my eyes automatically and effortlessly direct themselves toward her skin (are there spots?), her neck (is she moving it?), and her breathing (fast? slow? shallow?) even before her mother finishes describing the child's symptoms. When in top-down mode,

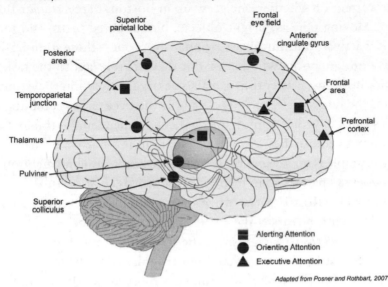

Some Components of the Three Attention Pathways

Superior parietal lobe

Frontal eye field

Anterior cingulate gyrus

Posterior area

Frontal area

Temporoparietal junction

Prefrontal cortex

Thalamus

Pulvinar

Superior colliculus

■ Alerting Attention
● Orienting Attention
▲ Executive Attention

Adapted from Posner and Rothbart, 2007

I decide what's important (making sure she doesn't have measles or meningitis or pneumonia), and I look and listen for it.[20] Neuroscientists have identified what seems to be the major top-down attention pathway in the brain, known as the dorsal frontoparietal network, which interprets information and guides decision making.

CIRCUIT BREAKERS

While top-down attention is initiated by our expectations and goals, "bottom-up" attention is stimulus driven. It is otherwise known as alerting attention because it maintains vigilance for the *unexpected.* You are driving to work along your usual route, and before you get to that familiar stop sign, a deer suddenly leaps into the road. Your foot reaches the brake before you even realize you're seeing a deer, and not a gorilla or a pedestrian. A surgeon notices red blood in the surgical field and slows down so that her attention can be directed to the bleeder; then she cauterizes it before proceeding.

Some bottom-up stimuli are universal and innate—they capture one's attention whether one grew up in Boston, Barcelona, or Borneo. Moving objects, bright objects, blood, bared teeth, and loud noises activate bottom-up attention in everyone—these stimuli steal away our attention, whether or not they are relevant to the task at hand. Bottom-up attention can also be triggered by internal stimuli from the body itself, such as a pain in the back or a grumbling in the stomach. Other stimuli are "salience dependent"—things that stand out because they are meaningful to us in some way. An everyday example is how we perk up when we hear our name mentioned at a cocktail party. Or, in medicine, the words *chest pressure*.

I saw Jane Rostro in the office—a woman in her seventies whom I've known for years. Like many older patients, she would bring several concerns to each visit, some trivial and some more serious. On this visit her list included hemorrhoids, an arthritic knee, and an itchy rash. Then she mentioned, almost as an afterthought, a funny sensation "right here" while climbing stairs, motioning with a broad gesture encompassing most of her chest and abdomen. It had been worsening over the past several days. A pressure, but not a pain. My attention was diverted by the words *pressure* and *climbing stairs* because of their salience—they might be indicators of angina, a potentially life-threatening situation. Not quite aware I was doing so, I suddenly demoted the itchy rash discourse and put myself on a new set of tracks in a different direction. Once I had made a bottom-up shift in focus, I switched back into top-down mode, now going through a sequence of questions asking about indicators of heart disease—short of breath? puffy legs? family history?—having completely abandoned the itchy rash.

When I told the emergency department about her impending arrival, I mentioned Mrs. Rostro's "chest pain," even though she had called it "pressure" and never used the word *chest*. Unwittingly, I filled in the blanks. I described her symptom to the nurse differently from the way Mrs. Rostro experienced and described it, perhaps because in medical school I learned a category of symptoms called *chest pain* and not *this funny sensation kinda around here*. And I know that *chest pain* tends to capture the attention of the emergency room staff and that the patient will be seen more quickly. If my bottom-up attention had been malfunctioning completely, had I persisted with her itchy rash and hemorrhoids and ignored her vague feeling that something was amiss, the outcome might not have been as good. She was found to have a blockage in her right coronary artery, which was stented, resulting in relief of her symptoms, perhaps saving her life.

Bottom-up attention activates several neural networks. One of those networks resides on the right side of the brain, the side most often associated with intuition, novelty, creativity, hunches, and artistic expression.[21] This makes sense because bottom-up attention is more impressionistic and intuitive. Bottom-up attention also involves the limbic system, which regulates emotions such as fear. Perhaps this is why people often struggle to explain why their attention gets redirected; I find myself saying, "Well, she just *looked* sick," and only later do I put together the pieces of what might have contributed to that impression (pale skin, shallow breathing, lying still). The *just looked sick* intuition, for me and other clinicians, is not innate; it is a product of experience and my ability to assimilate patterns over time. If you're not observant and have trouble educating your intuition, you'll become what educators Carl Bereiter and Marlene Scardamalia call an "experienced non-expert"—someone you wouldn't want to have as your doctor.[22]

By the time doctors finish medical school, certain signs and symptoms become incorporated as salient. They reliably elicit bottom-up responses—for example, if the patient mentions chest pain or has slurred speech, most doctors drop what they're doing and shift gears. Bottom-up attention tends to act like an "involuntary circuit breaker," quickly turning off a top-down process and diverting attention to something more immediate. Other equally important signs and symptoms *don't* trigger physicians' circuit breakers as consistently. Recently, a capable resident took me to see a patient, in his mid-fifties, who was receiving treatment for kidney cancer. The cancer was potentially curable. He was in the hospital because the chemotherapy was making him sick. He seemed a bit flat, perhaps despondent. This is not unusual for patients in the

27

hospital—no one likes being there and no one sleeps well. But then he said that he was thinking of taking early retirement.

I completely missed the salience of that patient's statement; in fact, when I discussed the case with the resident, I couldn't recall having heard it at all, nor did I register the patient's mood. I was totally focused on prescribing medications for pain and nausea. But for the resident, it sounded an alarm. The resident felt a sinking feeling, a sadness. He wondered whether this feeling was triggered by the patient—whether the patient might be depressed or even suicidal—which then tripped his internal circuit breaker and captured his attention. In fact, the patient *was* depressed. We referred him for psychotherapy and he responded well. The resident's ability to pick up on this signal was a direct result of his awareness of his own emotions—the heaviness he felt only grew stronger the more he talked with the patient. This particular resident had good teachers and role models who helped him learn how to be more sensitive to patients' depression. He used his own emotions to inform his care of the patient. But he was exceptional; not all clinicians would have picked up on these clues.[23]

THE INNER MANAGER

Bottom-up attention is capricious. *Any* fast-moving object or loud noise can act as a circuit breaker, even when it is a distraction. Think of what happens when an ambulance goes by while you're trying to have a conversation at a café—you lose your train of thought even though the ambulance's trajectory doesn't intersect yours. And some things should be circuit breakers but aren't. Bottom-up attention tends to fail when things change gradually—a kidney gradually turning blue, a slowly expanding mass, gradual weight loss, deepening depression.[24] Here, only clinicians who are exquisitely attuned to salient cues (such as Mr. Laszlo's night sweats) can see what is really there.

For doctors, electronic health records are one of the most potent circuit breakers. Nearly every time I prescribe a medication, for example, warnings about drug toxicity or drug interactions flash on the computer screen in lurid eye-catching colors, whether the potential for trouble is trivial or life threatening. I lose my train of thought and my gaze is now captured by the computer screen, and the patient is left waiting.[25] It's impossible to investigate all of the warnings in detail; trying to do so would keep the average doctor up past midnight. Barraged with these warnings, it is understandable why clinicians ignore many of them and how they can set the stage for other errors due to fatigue and distraction. Designers of these programs, adept at computer operating systems, clearly were not taking into account the limits of clinicians' inner operating systems.

Executive attention is our "inner manager," which helps us to prioritize one source of information over another. Consider what happens when Mrs. Rostro returns to talking about her itchy rash. My attention is divided between the signs and symptoms of heart disease and the signs and symptoms of eczema, far less serious. If it's a normal day in the office, my visit with Mrs. Rostro might be interrupted by a knock on the door from my nurse, who informs me that the last prescription I wrote for a different patient is not covered by his insurance. I look at my mobile phone to find the phone number for the cardiologist to call regarding Mrs. Rostro, and I note a calendar alert to bring the car in for an oil change. When I hear the distant sound of a car alarm, which I'd usually ignore, I realize that I'd forgotten to bring the car in for the oil change. I sniffle, then become aware that I'm still fatigued, just having gotten over a cold. Executive attention triages stimuli and in the best of circumstances helps me pay attention to what matters— Mrs. Rostro's concerns—and to ignore the rest.

TWENTY MINUTES OF RED

When I was in college in the 1970s, I took a course with Ken Maue, a visionary avant-garde musician. Ken wanted his musicians to experience beauty and harmony by inviting them to see the world differently, in unexpected and surprising ways. He composed a performance piece that was originally intended to last three days—hence the original title, *Three Days of Red*.[26]

The instructions are simple: "For three days record in writing everything red that you see." I actually did it once, back in 1973. Although the act of "seeing red" for three consecutive days for me was life changing (I could never again see the world in the same way), even a few minutes can be instructive (and far more pragmatic). You're instructed to spend twenty minutes (or as long as an hour or as short as seven minutes) walking in the environment (often a hospital or conference center) in silence. I also ask you to notice what's going on in your own mind during the exercise. This exercise directs your top-down, goal-directed attention to things red. While you're observing your reactions, the exercise helps you be more aware of your inner experience, such as bottom-up impressions, emotions, and thoughts that enter your awareness. You might want to stop here and try it.

Twenty Minutes of Red

For the next twenty minutes,
record in writing the name
of everything red that you see.

The red exercise leads participants to realize that there is no "immaculate perception"—we don't see things as they are as much as we see things as conditioned by our expectations and goals.[27] People doing the exercise are frequently surprised at how many red things they now notice that had previously escaped their attention—even in a familiar environment. They ask themselves, "How red does something need to be to be called red?" They discern finer gradations of red, purple, orange, and pink. Some get competitive and try to list more red things, and more unusual red things, than their colleagues. Some get bored, some get excited, some get annoyed, and some worry if they're doing the exercise correctly—all of these thoughts and feelings bubble up unbidden from their bottom-up attention.

One of the reasons people find the red exercise so compelling is that they learn how their minds work; nearly all of them note that anything that is not red tends to be discounted. They literally see the world differently, and they see how inputs from the senses are filtered by their brains before they are apprehended as conscious perceptions. The red objects were always there, but now we notice them and notice how we notice them. It lays mental processes—normally in the background—in plain sight. These mental processes not only filter information that happens to come our way, they also drive our own information-seeking behaviors—we look, seek out, and even redefine objects as red.

The red exercise has its counterparts in medicine. It's common for medical students taking a dermatology rotation to begin to notice every freckle on each passerby. They might be more aware of the different brands of sunscreen on display when they go to the supermarket. During flu season, I see dozens of patients with influenza. I begin to divide the world of patients with respiratory symptoms into "flu" and "not flu." I wonder how "flu-like" the patient's symptoms need to be to consider it a case of flu—and not another respiratory virus or a bacterial pneumonia that would require antibiotics.

But clinical medicine is more complex than simple pattern recognition; we not only see patterns, we enact *scripts*.[28] In the emergency room, when an overweight middle-aged woman describes severe pain in the right upper quadrant of the abdomen, a physician's "gallbladder script" is activated. The physician's top-down attention is directed to listen for symptoms of pain and nausea after eating fatty foods, to consider whether a radiologist is available to interpret an ultrasound of the gallbladder, and to prepare to order intravenous fluids and pain relievers. This all happens in an instant.

But scripts aren't always reliable. For most physicians, the gallbladder script would be triggered by someone who has recently eaten a fatty meal and reinforced if the patient is "fair, fat, fertile, female over forty"—the five F's mnemonic that medical students use to recall features of typical patients with biliary colic, the pain that occurs when a gallstone gets stuck, blocking the exit of bile.

While this script would readily identify the "typical" patient, the majority of patients with biliary colic do not have all of these clinical features; if they've not eaten a fatty meal or if they are black, male, young, or thin, the physician typically takes longer to consider gallbladder disease. Or, conversely, patients with the five F's might not have a gallbladder problem at all—they may have had too much to drink or have heartburn. By assuming that upper abdominal pain is due to gallbladder disease, the physician might not think to ask about other symptoms, such as shortness of breath, that might suggest something far more ominous (a heart attack). The same mental scripts that are helpful and efficient in straightforward situations can prevent us from seeing what is actually there in more complex ones.[29]

The red exercise also has its counterpart in human relationships. If a doctor (or anyone else) has a preconceived idea about others— for example, their intelligence, the legitimacy of their symptoms, or their truthfulness—he will tend to discount evidence to the contrary. The effects of these expectations are even more powerful if the physician harbors unexamined negative emotions such as dislike, fear, guilt, anger, disgust, or annoyance.[30]

Those expectations sometimes affect clinical care. I had a close call several years ago. Patricia Scarpa, a middle-aged woman whom I knew well, did not come to the clinic often, but when she came, it always took a long time. She usually had a litany of aches and pains for which no cause could be found. She was not particularly distressed or depressed; this was just the way she was. Her voice was whiny, and she would elaborate in great detail about each item in her list of symptoms. As much as I tried to be attentive, after a while I couldn't focus. I'd get impatient and annoyed.

On this particular visit, she mentioned worsening vague belly pain and bloating, not severe but noticeable. Finding nothing on her physical exam, I relegated this symptom to another one of her uncomfortable but nonserious concerns for which I could only hope to offer some empathy, reassurance, and symptom relief— and did. Later that evening, when I was completing my notes, my eye darted to the vital-signs portion of her chart. She hadn't mentioned it, but she had lost nearly fifteen pounds since her last visit. The next day I called her and asked how she was doing. No better. I suggested that she come back in a few days. That time, I did a more careful physical exam, worried that she might have cancer. Although it was subtle, I thought I could feel fluid in her belly, not a normal thing. I hadn't scheduled the time for a gynecologic exam, but I took the time to do it—and found a hard mass that proved to be ovarian cancer. Had I not called her in, or if I'd felt rushed or inattentive, the opportunity for a cure might have been lost.[31]

WHAT MINDFUL ATTENTION LOOKS LIKE

A colleague, a seasoned neurologist, greets a new patient. Watching the patient extend his hand for a handshake, something attracts the neurologist's attention, something subtle in the patient's movement—something that would not be noticed by a layperson. She cannot name that "something," yet it triggers the thought "Watch out, be attentive, something is amiss." The patient, previously thought to have Parkinson's disease, just doesn't have the type of hesitancy and difficulty initiating movements that would be expected if he did have Parkinson's. Ultimately the patient is diagnosed with a small stroke, which prompts a different approach to treatment; the neurologist stops the potentially toxic medications for Parkinson's and starts blood thinners to prevent another stroke.

My hunch is that this neurologist—like other master clinicians— uses her whole mind to a greater degree than her less skilled counterparts. Master clinicians attend to the person in front of them while attending to their own mental processes. They don't take for granted their initial impressions, or anyone else's. They attend to that which they can explicitly describe, as well as the vague impressions that influence their judgment. They use their analytic minds— knowledge, evidence, and technical skills—as well as their intuitive and imaginative minds, the sensibilities that we typically associate with the humanities.[32]

What does focused attention feel like? For an experienced cyclist, focused attention means maintaining balance while going around a sharp curve. For a musician, it is making exquisite each brief silence between two notes. For a surgeon, it is applying just the right amount of tension to a suture. For a neurologist, it is knowing when to let a first impression guide your thinking and when those impressions lead you astray. Attending in this way is the result of more than just experience. It takes practice to bring perceptions to awareness when needed, and to allow them to fade below the threshold of awareness at other times to avoid overloading the mental circuits,[33] employing all three kinds of attention to perceive and respond to that which might otherwise have been missed.

Applying focused attention is a *moral* choice, not just a skill. We pay attention to that which we consider important, and by virtue of paying attention to something, we make it important. All physicians take a vow to do their best to relieve suffering and not do harm. But unknowingly, sometimes we attend to some kinds of suffering—and some people who suffer—more than others. Attending to each patient's concerns means more than just becoming more perceptive and attentive; it means being prepared to greet whatever concerns patients bring with curiosity and resolve.

3

Curiosity

The sixty-year-old man lay motionless, and the whooshing sound of the ventilator was the only thing that broke the late-night still- ness. He had had a large stroke and his condition hadn't changed during the five days he had been in the hospital. His family was dis- traught; each day they came in and talked to him, rubbed his hand, wiped his face, desperately trying to establish contact, to see if he could respond in any way. Nothing. Then came their tears. On day number four, I was told, one family member thought that she saw him blink one eye in response to a question; otherwise he was flick- erless. He had electrodes on his head for continuous EEG monitor- ing. The brain waves were normal, meaning that most likely he was "locked in"—able to think, but not able to move or respond in any way, a terrifying prospect. That morning, we rounded quickly. Still no change, no communication, zero. The intern wrote in the chart, "Unresponsive; prognosis poor."

I was still at the hospital late at night and I had just finished my notes. I peered into the patient's darkened room and was surprised to see Dr. Fisher. I was a medical student, fortunate to have been assigned to a renowned senior neurologist, C. Miller Fisher, for a month-long rotation. Fisher was an observant and thoughtful man, but I saw him doing things in the room that struck me as, well, odd. Flashlight in hand, he illuminated parts of the room, then shone it on his own face while talking to the patient, gesticulating wildly and making grotesque facial expressions—sneers, grins, frowns— almost clownlike. Then he'd stop and check the EEG machine for any spike in the visual cortex or the auditory cortex when he was talking and gesticulating—hoping to see what was still working in the patient's brain and to connect in some way with the patient as a person. Fisher assumed that the patient had an inner life and wanted to see if he was capable of a two-way connection with the world. He assumed that "unresponsive" merely meant that he had not found the correct channels for communication. Fisher didn't know what he would find. Ultimately, he noted a flicker of movement around the patient's eyes, just like what the family had described. Fisher noted a simultaneous EEG spike in the visual cortex—confirming the family's impressions that the message was getting through. The patient, otherwise barely showing signs of life, was responding. We communicated this news to the family the next day. Even though we will never know what impact that human gesture had on the patient—his ability to communicate never improved—the family found solace knowing that their messages of love and caring were getting through.

Fisher's curiosity was palpable. Like the late Oliver Sacks, he had perfected the art and joy of observation. Like others who are curious, his gratification was intrinsic; when being curious, we explore new things for their own sake with no extrinsic reward.[1] Inevitably, this kind of exploration yields unexpected surprises.

Curiosity is a fundamental human quality and is essential for survival; during a famine, those who seek out novel sources of food and shelter are likely to fare better (Who would imagine that the inside of a prickly thistle could be a delicacy or that cold slippery ice could be made into a warm cozy igloo?). Curiosity is "wonderment,"[2] a realization that there is always more; personality researchers consider curiosity a manifestation of a psychological trait, "openness to experience."[3] In medicine, curiosity means seeking to know what makes each person tick. An attraction to the unknown, the unusual, and the unexpected is also what makes great physician-scientists. Whereas most scientists were throwing away moldy petri dishes, Alexander Fleming, an inquisitive but otherwise undistinguished scientist, discovered the mold that would be synthesized into penicillin.

Throughout medical school, residency, and clinical practice, doctors are socialized to be authoritative, knowledgeable, and self-confident. Saying "I don't know" is not an option. Perhaps curiosity is seen as immature or even dangerous. Students' probing questions—a sign of curiosity—are not always well received by supervising physicians.

Curiosity is sidelined by what Jerome Kassirer, former editor of the *New England Journal of Medicine*, called a "stubborn quest for certainty." Being too certain—never being in doubt—paradoxically results in lower-quality care through overtesting, premature conclusions, and tunnel vision.[4] Psychologically, when doctors (or anyone else) are barraged with information and in a hurry, we find it harder to be curious, to explore outside the box, to entertain doubt. The pressure to solve problems quickly leads doctors to rely on rules and mental shortcuts rather than to consider each situation afresh. In their more mindless moments, doctors do tests "just to be sure," then abandon their curiosity when a test confirms their initial impressions. Content with a solution that is expedient and not necessarily optimal, they don't explore a full range of options. They tacitly assume that being open or curious takes too much time and energy, not recognizing that putting on blinders will cost them time later. In a word, they *satisfice*.

Faith Fitzgerald's 1999 essay on curiosity should be required reading for all health professionals.[5] An internist, Fitzgerald was dean of students at the University of California, Davis, School of Medicine. Typically, on rounds, senior physicians ask trainees to present the most interesting patients admitted overnight. *Interesting*—in medical discourse—is code for rare diseases (usually incurable) or atypical manifestations of more common ones, things that are easy to miss. Or, sometimes, a "classic" presentation of a serious disease—the loud murmur signaling a ruptured heart valve or bruises on the abdomen signaling severe pancreatitis. *Interesting* is in contrast to the typical day, which for most clinicians is filled with things that, on the surface, seem quite ordinary; for cardiologists it's chest pain, for neurologists it's headache, for dermatologists it's acne. Fitzgerald, in a brilliant educational exercise, would turn the question on its head; she would ask residents to present their most *boring* patient. Her goal was to promote curiosity by demonstrating that every patient's story was unique, interesting, and vital to her care.

One morning, the residents picked an elderly woman who was admitted for "social" reasons: she had been evicted from her apartment, had nowhere to go, and showed up at the hospital emergency room, destitute and confused, with little in the way of medical illness. Her answers to questions were monosyllabic. Her medical history was sparse, her family was gone, and she seemed to have no interests. Fitzgerald wasn't getting anywhere. Finally she asked the patient if she had ever been hospitalized.

"Yes, I broke my arm," she said.

"How did that happen?"

"A steamer trunk fell on it."

Fitzgerald persisted; answers slowly unfolded. The patient was emigrating from Ireland to the United States. The boat lurched. It had hit an iceberg. The name of the boat—you guessed it.[6] In the same essay, Fitzgerald told another story about a resident who noted a scar in a patient's groin. The patient said that he had been bitten by a snake there. "How did that happen?" Fitzgerald asked. The resident said he didn't know. As Fitzgerald noted, the imagination can run riot with possibilities.

While Fitzgerald's stories relate to knowing the patient as a person, curiosity is also essential to the technical aspects of care. Several years ago, on my first day of a much-needed vacation, I was trying to unstick the quick-release lever on a bicycle seat post. The lever snapped and the rusty broken end impaled the muscle at the base of my left thumb. It was a deep wound. After stitches and a week for the swelling to go down, I still had numbness on the outside (radial side) of the thumb. The hand surgeon explained to his resident (and me) that nerve injury on the radial side of the thumb was less important than on the ulnar side of the thumb because the ulnar side was needed for a pincer grasp—turning screws and handling instruments. Thus, they would not plan any further tests or interventions. They didn't think to ask what I actually do with my hands. For me, doing physical examinations, typing on a computer, and playing the harpsichord are everyday activities that require sensation on the radial side of the thumb. I rarely use a pen, a screwdriver, or a scalpel. As an assertive patient, I objected. They changed their plan and, fortunately, the numbness resolved.

In medicine, feeling not-too-certain leads good clinicians to dig further, to explore the archaeology of each person's illness. Social psychologist Ellen Langer recommends that we consider "facts" as merely provisional or contextual—what's true today in Rochester, New York, might not be true tomorrow—or elsewhere. Facts come to us from our primary senses ("I saw it with my own eyes," etc.) and also through spoken or written language. Any trial lawyer or astute clinician knows better than to accept these primary data as irrevocably true.

Faith Fitzgerald, in her article on curiosity, tells a story of a medical student who presents a patient on rounds as having "BKA times two." In medical jargon, BKA stands for "below-the-knee amputation." Fitzgerald saw the patient and noted two feet sticking out from under the sheets—warm, pink, hairy. Even seeing the patient with Dr. Fitzgerald, the student failed to notice that the patient had feet until she pointed it out. The student was flummoxed, rendered speechless. He said that he reported BKA because it said so in the chart. Apparently, a transcriptionist made an error on a discharge summary. Instead of typing DKA (diabetic ketoacidosis), she typed BKA. The error was carried through several hospital admissions. Once a patient is assigned a diagnosis, whether it be a disease (asthma, for example) or a personal characteristic (e.g., "difficult," "noncompliant"), that diagnosis tends to stick, and it takes what seems like an act of Congress to remove it from the patient's profile.[7] It shuts down consideration of alternatives.

In medicine, curiosity about people is not merely a nicety. A spirit of inquiry, interest, and wonder is good for patients—and fundamental to excellent care—because clinicians then see them in all of their richness and complexity. Adopting an attitude of being not quite certain can release clinicians from the tyranny of categories, or at least soften their edges. They see patients as humans, not merely case studies. Curiosity can help clinicians choose the right treatment; asking someone how he spends his day can help me know whether taking a pill three times a day is realistic or if a once-daily dosing (at slightly higher cost) is better. A deep interest in people is the basis for empathy and understanding. Curiosity, like attention, has a moral dimension: it inspires care that respects and engages with patients' needs, wants, preferences, and values.[8]

FUZZY TRACES

In primary care practice, patients typically present with early and subtle signs of illness, making a diagnosis more difficult. Appendicitis in its early stages can seem just like an ordinary stomachache. Pneumonia and heart failure may be hard to distinguish from one another. An allergic reaction and a staph skin infection may look alike. Some diseases have early signs and symptoms that are just too subtle to detect, but are obvious in retrospect. Sometimes it doesn't matter if the diagnosis is delayed, but at other times an early diagnosis is critical.

As a family physician, I see many children in my office with cold symptoms, often the victims of some virus. However, every once in a while, a child with symptoms similar to those of a virus has something more serious—pneumonia, meningitis, even leukemia. In those situations, often something doesn't feel quite right to me. I feel a sense of unease. My brain is on high alert, yet the accompanying feelings are visceral and hard to describe—I just don't feel comfortable inside. Sometimes I wake up in the middle of the night, worried. Perhaps I told a mother to bring her child back in a week; now that seems too long. These visceral feelings draw upon and also inform what philosopher Michael Polanyi calls "tacit knowledge"[9] (that which we know but find difficult to describe) and what psychologist Valerie Reyna calls "fuzzy traces" (memories that carry the gist of a situation but are often fuzzy about details).[10]

What happens next is particularly important; it would be so easy to ignore the feeling and move along to the next task. But I'm curious when a patient "looks sick." I can explore it, unpack it, and examine it more closely. Perhaps the child is a bit pale or is clinging to his mother more than I'd expect. Perhaps I know that his mother doesn't schedule office visits unless something is really wrong—and she's usually on the mark.

When being curious, this sense of unease piques my interest in the patient. I am attuned in a way that invites further exploration, often before I can characterize why—perhaps in the same way that a sommelier can first identify a great wine and only later finds the adjectives to describe it. Clearly, these impressions are informed by my clinical expertise; I would not have been able to make fine distinctions between "sick" and "really sick" prior to having gone to medical school, just as a sommelier needs to have learned a vocabulary to distinguish different types of grapes and styles of winemaking. From discernment comes curiosity, and then greater discernment. Curiosity is more than mere experience; it links heightened attention ("Something's not quite right") with self-awareness ("I'm feeling uncomfortable"), knowledge ("This situation could be dangerous"), and exploration ("I wonder what's going on").[11]

A BAD DAY

Curiosity suffers when we feel befuddled and besieged. Alexis Brown and I had met just once before, not quite three weeks earlier, shortly after she had been hospitalized with a myocardial infarction—a heart attack. Alexis was only forty-two years old and had considered herself healthy and fit. Today she was scheduled for a complete physical.

The visit started with an initial greeting and a general inquiry about her concerns.

"Things are okay."

"How do you feel you've been recovering since the heart attack?" I asked.

"I didn't have a heart attack."

I was taken aback. "I don't understand. I thought we'd gone over that."

"They did the first test and it was normal, then a few hours later they told me it was abnormal. Then they told me there was no blockage."

Suddenly, doubting my memory, I paused. "Could I check the note your cardiologist wrote?" I wanted to be certain, beyond doubt.

I found the note from the cardiologist. Sure enough, the EKG tracing showed ST-wave changes characteristic of a myocardial infarction. The blood troponin levels were initially normal, then elevated four hours later, indicating heart damage. So far, pretty typical for a heart attack. Her cardiac catheterization didn't reveal fixed blockages in any of her coronary arteries. This was unusual, surprising. However, the right coronary artery went into spasm during the test, transiently blocking blood flow—a characteristic of Prinzmetal's syndrome, an uncommon condition and even more rarely a cause of a heart attack. My notes indicated that I had discussed all of this with Ms. Brown the last time and she had seemed to understand. I was sure I was right. But now, it was as if the prior discussion hadn't occurred.

I asked about exercise.

"I'm not exercising."

"Why is that?"

"They never told me what I could do to prevent this from happening again."

"And medication? I see that they prescribed lisinopril and metoprolol to prevent future heart damage."

"I read the side effects and I'm not taking them."

I was growing annoyed, frustrated. We reviewed her lab tests. Cholesterol good. Stopped smoking in the hospital, none since. Doesn't drink. I tried to plow through.

"So, maybe we should do the physical exam. Here's a gown; I'll be back in about two minutes.

"I don't think I want a physical today."

"Okay, we can wait if you like. I was reviewing your chart and noticed that you don't have a flu shot on record. Can I offer you one?"

A hesitation. "No, I don't think I want it."

"Can I ask why?"

"I don't think I will get the flu."

The more she protested, the more I pushed, offering things, services and recommendations. I had no interest in why she might be acting the way she was.

"I just don't want it," she said.

Now I felt under attack. I thought, "Why the hell is she coming in today, anyway? To torment me?" I was running late already and had no patience for what I perceived as stonewalling.

Perhaps you see this situation more clearly than I did at the time. I didn't welcome her perspective. I was impatient with her lack of cooperation, not seeing that my impatience was the flip side of my need to be an authority, in charge. I just wanted to push ahead with my agenda and get this increasingly unpleasant visit over with. She had seemed so reasonable during our first visit, and now this. To reassert control I started on a quiet rampage, "I thought that we agreed that you'd come in for complete—" Not being able to finish my own sentence, I stopped abruptly. An awkward silence.

Then, I smiled at myself. I realized that *she* was not making me annoyed, that *my own mind* was creating this sense of annoyance because I desired something (a docile, agreeable patient) that was not in the offing. Call this a mindful moment. I realized, with a calm equanimity, that I was trying to push her into compliance and that I was serving my own need to have the visit follow a particular protocol. My breathing had become shallow and I had an almost insatiable desire to sigh. I had been tensing my legs as if preparing to bolt. I wanted to get out of there. I hadn't been curious about how Alexis Brown saw the situation nor about what she felt she needed. I had had no interest in examining my contribution to— and her experience of—our breakdown in communication.

Here, the sense of unease finally roused my curiosity. I inquired, not having any idea how she might respond, "Can I ask you, how are we doing here? I'm not sure what you were hoping for today."

"We're doing okay."

There was another silence, this time less awkward and more expectant.

"I'm the one who's in control here. I know my body and I don't need a physical."

"That's really important. You want to be in control. I understand that to mean you want to know what's going on so that you can be in charge of your health. Is that right?"

"Yes." We had arrived somewhere. She had a few questions, all germane to her illness and its treatment. I still felt uncomfortable.

"So how should we leave things? Normally I'd see someone back a couple of times in the first few weeks after a hospitalization, but it's up to you. You could come back in a week, a month . . ." I expected her to say that she'd call when she needed to and that I'd never see her again.

"How about two weeks."

I was stunned.

"You're the first doctor who explained things."

"I'll try, but you let me know when we go off course." I meant it; I did need her help.

"Okay, see you then."

The next week a note from the cardiologist indicated that she was doing well and was content taking her medications.

TRAVELING IN PACKS AND PRACTICING ALONE

While curiosity is often spontaneous, sometimes it takes effort, especially when things aren't going well. As communication was breaking down with Ms. Brown, I didn't *want* to be curious; I just wanted to get out of there. Physiologically, the stress of conflict activated my three-way fight-or-flight-or-freeze switch—not my curiosity switch. I wanted to place the responsibility and blame for malfunctioning communication on her. How easy it would be to say that she was "in denial" or "noncompliant," leaving a fractured relationship unaddressed and a serious disease untreated. I needed a way of bringing myself back to the present, to engage with her in a more productive way. This took an additional minute or two of time and some additional mental effort, but likely saved me hours down the road.

I tried to dissect what had happened. As I became aware that my breathing was shallow and that I had been tensing my legs, I had a "fuzzy trace" moment—something was amiss but I couldn't put my finger on it. I then noticed the associated emotions—feelings of restlessness and frustration. At first I tried to push those sensations and emotions away, then realized that they were a useful signal. What I was doing wasn't working, and the clue came from feelings in my body. I listened to the signals coming from within and used those signals as triggers to become *more* curious, to slow down and inquire further, even though I was feeling annoyed. While it could have happened sooner (I became curious after having tried several other options!), this subtle transition was instrumental in achieving a positive outcome.

Achieving a transition like that—transforming discomfort into curiosity—takes practice, both in the clinic and outside. One exercise that can be particularly useful is the "body scan," popularized by Jon Kabat-Zinn in his Mindfulness-Based Stress Reduction programs. The body scan is not a relaxation exercise; rather, it's an awareness exercise.[12] Participants are guided through awareness of each part of the body, noting its position in space, tension, relaxation, or other pleasant or unpleasant sensations. When "scanning" the abdomen and chest, the attention is drawn to movement—of the breath, the viscera, and the heart. Sometimes I'll experience a strange sense of unfamiliarity and novelty—for example, when I first noticed that I habitually hold my left shoulder more hunched than the right. Simply noticing and exploring bodily sensations—without trying to change them—lets you observe more fully. Paradoxically, practiced inaction can lead to action. In the clinic that day, a brief taste of that practiced awareness was essential in switching from frustration to inquiry.

Well-functioning clinical teams can also promote curiosity. A palliative care nurse-practitioner colleague routinely explains to patients when we arrive with a group, all in white coats, "We travel in packs for protection."[13] While it's an attempt to make humor out of a potentially threatening situation, there is some truth in it. Several sets of eyes and ears, in a well-functioning team, extend the senses and sensibilities of any one individual. A team member might say, "Did you notice she's looking a bit yellow?" or "She seems to be more confused today than yesterday," or "I don't think that we're all on the same page." A new observation then leads to doubt, reconsideration, and revision of our impressions. Observant teams stimulate an infectious curiosity.

However, as clinicians, we often practice alone. Even in the hospital, after rounds, I visit patients by myself. In my family medicine office, a patient arrives and the door is shut. It's just me and the patient—and possibly a family member or two. No one is watching. Almost no one has directly observed my practice in thirty years—except the occasional medical student. In those situations, curiosity has to start with me. If I'm being mindful, I am curious about the patient and I am curious about my own experience. In a way that is informative and not self-indulgent, I notice what captures my attention as I go about my work, whether I find it pleasant or unpleasant, interesting or annoying. I am "preparing to be unprepared"; I practice what Ellen Langer calls "soft vigilance," an open, receptive awareness, actively looking for something that is new, unexpected, or interesting.[14] Soft vigilance is a relaxed awareness. It is different from hypervigilance—trying to focus on every detail at every moment. Soft vigilance is energizing, whereas hypervigilance can be exhausting. Soft vigilance informs and prepares me to pay attention in a different, more open way.

PURSUING DOUBT

If curiosity is its own reward, one would expect that people—including doctors—would display it more often. Yet being curious also takes people outside their comfort zones because it has to do with *increasing*—not removing—uncertainty. It goes counter to the human tendency to oblige reality to fit our preconceived notions. Being curious involves being aware that the situation is not as tidy as it might seem. This sense of doubt is unsettling for many doctors and patients, especially when the stakes are high.[15] Patients undergoing surgery for cancer want to hear—and surgeons want to say—"I got it all." Patients and doctors want a diagnosis to be definitive, beyond doubt, and a treatment to be the best available. Sometimes we have that degree of certainty, but more often that certainty is elusive—provisional, incomplete, or evolving. While a biopsy can prove that you have cancer, it cannot tell you exactly how long you will live or if you will be the one who will benefit from treatment or the one who won't. Being mindful means *feeling* uncertainty, *not turning away from* that feeling of uncertainty and *not clinging to* the negative emotions that arise.[16]

Curiosity not only draws attention to the outside world, but also draws attention to one's inner experience: "Am I tired? Am I too sure of myself? Am I in a hurry? What's new here?" Even the way clinicians interact with patients can help them be curious: "I'm wondering—have I addressed what's really important to you? Am I missing something? Is there something more that you want to tell me?" I make a habit of asking myself "What's interesting about this patient?" and "What's still unknown?" as a habitual (but not foolproof) way of avoiding self-deception and premature closure.

Curiosity is not only good for patient care; it is also good for health professionals. By enriching their connections with their patients and feeling more effective—on their game—they feel more vitality in their work.[17] Recent research suggests that there's a feedback loop between curiosity on the one hand, and anxiety, defensiveness, and rigidity on the other. For years, psychologists have known (mostly from research in educational settings) that when we're less anxious, defensive, and rigid, curiosity flourishes. New research suggests that it also works the other way; the more curious you are, the less anxious, defensive, and rigid you'll be when under psychological stress. Psychologist Todd Kashdan conducted an interesting set of experiments in which participants were asked to think about their death, imagining what a terminal illness and dying might be like. As predicted by "terror management theory" (and common sense), subjects became defensive; they tried to push away death-related thoughts and tended to cling to familiar beliefs, people, and surroundings. The researchers also measured attentiveness and curiosity, both elements of mindfulness. People who were attentive and curious were less anxious and defensive than those who were equally attentive but had a less curious disposition.[18]

Some people have personalities that seek novelty; they tend to be adventurous and less risk-averse. They see new challenges as exciting rather than terrifying. These tendencies manifest early in childhood, leading to speculation that brain chemistry, genetics, and social environment might all contribute.[19] Curiosity is associated with release of the neurotransmitter dopamine, activating intrinsic reward circuits in the brain.[20] These dopaminergic systems are triggered by novel experiences, especially sensory experiences, and magnified if the experiences are surprising and associated with some risk (Think about adolescents here!). Because dopamine release makes one feel good, curiosity persists even in the absence of tangible external rewards. People who score high on psychological markers of curiosity—in particular, those who have high "openness"—are biochemically different from their peers. Their dopamine receptors are more numerous and their genetic controlling mechanisms are different.[21] The propensity to be curious is, to some degree, encoded on our genes.[22]

Curiosity is not merely genetic; it grows in nurturing social environments. Children's "exploration behaviors"—analogous to the more critical and nuanced curiosity of adults—are expressed to a greater degree among children whose emotional attachment to their parents and other adults is secure. Children raised in a supportive environment feel safer taking small risks and exploring the unknown than children who have experienced less nurturance. For them, curiosity leads to a sense of vividness—children feel that their world "comes alive" and provides a sense of fulfillment and happiness.[23] They want to explore further, widening their reach. In contrast, those raised in abusive or neglectful environments tend to adopt a more fearful, anxious, or avoidant attachment style and cling to the familiar.[24] They don't explore or examine the world around them. They're afraid of rejection and failure. When they become adults, the same factors hold true. Like children, adults are more curious in supportive environments—ones that promote inquiry and in which they can safely share their doubts, discoveries, and mishaps.[25] Yet, clinicians tend to rate their work environments as not particularly supportive. They often rely on the relationships that they develop outside the workplace for support.[26]

While in the past the social/cognitive environment and genetics were seen as opposing explanations for human behavior, the relatively new—and exciting—fields of behavioral and social epigenetics have made clear that the social environment affects the ways in which one's genetic predispositions are actually expressed.[27] If the social environment is safe and supportive, the genes that encode dopamine receptors are turned on. With more receptors, the sense of intrinsic reward from discovery and curiosity is greater. Conversely, if the environment is abusive or inconsistent, the same genes will be turned off. Put simply, genes affect psychological states and social interactions, and also the reverse—these same genes are regulated by the internal psychological environment as well as the social milieu. Even those who might have a low "natural" tendency toward curiosity become more curious if placed in a supportive environment with strong healthy relationships and encouragement to reflect and be self-aware.

Curiosity is part of the social capital of medicine. Just like young children, medical practitioners who are more curious feel a greater sense of vividness and vitality. They are more satisfied with their work, more engaged with their patients, and do a better job of treating illnesses. Entertain, for a moment, the radical thought that health care institutions could actually support healthy learning environments. Clinicians would be more motivated; they'd inquire more deeply about patients' illnesses and distress, form more meaningful relationships, and have a greater sense of self-confidence—all of which would promote greater quality of care.

4

Beginner's Mind

The Zen of Doctoring

When I was nineteen, I spent three months at the San Francisco Zen Center. I had read a book, *Zen Mind, Beginner's Mind*, written by Shunryu Suzuki Roshi, the founding abbot of the center. Shortly thereafter I applied to be a "guest student." In the book, Suzuki Roshi describes in simple language the core principles of mindful living and meditation practice.[1] It's one of my "stranded on a desert island" books—each time I pick up the small volume, I find new wisdom. Suzuki Roshi said, "In the beginner's mind the possibilities are many, in the expert's they are few." By this he meant that expertise can lead you to deep insights, but can also lead your mind away from its true nature—curious, open, creative.[2] At that time I was a beginner, so I found this reassuring. But beginner's mind is even more important for those with some claim to expertise.

During one of my medical school rotations, a classmate was assigned a patient with hairy-cell leukemia, a disease that was fascinating to the physicians caring for her because the genetic basis of the disease had recently been discovered. (It's called "hairy" because of the appearance of the cells under the microscope.) She was considered a "great case." Despite our exquisite understanding of her illness, the treatments available provided no guarantees of a cure. On rounds with my classmate and our supervising residents, I saw a frail woman, bedridden, without family or get-well cards in her room. No one seemed to be addressing either her pain or her isolation. It didn't take much—my classmate took a moment to mention to the clinical team that the patient seemed uncomfortable and alone. Once alerted, the team provided a different kind of attention, focused on comfort and dignity; they ordered pain medications and arranged for a chaplain to come to the bedside. My classmate's supervisor, clearly more expert than he, saw her as a "great case"; it took a beginner's eyes to see her as a "suffering person."

Now that I am the senior member of clinical teams, I value medical students' input more than ever. Often the medical student on the team is the one who asks the key question—something as simple as "Why are you doing *that*?" The naïve (and sometimes annoying!) questions of a bright medical student can profoundly alter an experienced clinician's point of view. Recently a medical student asked me whether our social worker could help with transportation for an elderly patient with diabetes. Until he asked, I hadn't considered *why* the patient had missed so many appointments; turns out she had no reliable way of getting to the office, and that's why her diabetes was out of control. In retrospect it seems so obvious.

When Suzuki Roshi talked about beginner's mind, he was talking to (or about) beginners, but his message was even more important for experts. Experts tenaciously hold on to their expertise. They conflate their competence and experience with mastery. After all, we have worked hard to become the experts that we are, and suggesting that this hard-earned expertise should be set aside is a radical notion. But experts don't always see how their expertise can limit their understanding. In the view of the Dreyfus brothers, professors at the University of California, Berkeley, who developed a model of expertise, experts know the answers, but only masters know the important questions. Experts revel in what they know, and masters revel in what they don't.[3]

Expertise can lead doctors to assume that they know things that they cannot. For example, doctors often feel that they are able to assess patients' pain accurately. Patients' accounts (backed up by research) suggest otherwise, that we don't really know much about our patients' distress unless we ask. Physicians' estimates about their patients' level of pain are often no better than chance, meaning that we often provide inadequate (or unnecessarily excessive) pain medication. Psychologist Cleve Shields studies communication between patients and physicians. He read transcripts of audio-recorded patient-physician office visits in which there was some discussion of pain. Physicians who used more "certainty words"—words that connoted that they were sure of themselves, beyond doubt—asked patients fewer questions about their pain: what it was like, what helped and what didn't. The doctors' presumptuousness got in the way of good care.[4] Doctors, as they go through training, often get worse at understanding patients' subjective experience of illness; the doctors' expertise blinds them to patients' experience of suffering and their empathy declines.[5] They give privilege to objective information *about* patients over subjective information *from* patients. They are more likely to treat patients as diagnoses, as objects. Neuroimaging studies suggest that physicians are less emotionally reactive to seeing patients in pain than the general population—a good thing because it keeps them from becoming overwhelmed, a bad thing because sometimes they objectify patients and distance themselves too much.[6]

Beginner's mind uncouples expertise from one's present experience. It is a cultivated naïveté, an intentional setting aside of the knowledge and preconceived notions that one has gained from books, journals, teachers, and past experiences to see the situation with new eyes. I think of it as putting my "expert self" on an imaginary shelf for a moment, easily within reach and readily available, but enough out of the way so that it doesn't become an encumbrance to a more intuitive and holistic way of being. I think, "What does this patient need most today?" Then I seek the evidence to justify or refute my initial impressions. Simply setting my expert self aside helps me to consider new possibilities.

Johann Sebastian Bach is reported to have said, "The problem is not finding [melodies], it's—when getting up in the morning and out of bed—not stepping on them."[7] Bach was a consummate expert, perhaps the greatest composer who ever lived, and was continually creative and inventive within a tradition that had strict rules of composition. However, to be creative, he had to set aside some of his preconceived notions of what music could be to produce something new, fresh, and not formulaic. The same was true of other great composers who created new musical languages: Monteverdi, Beethoven, Wagner, Schönberg, and Cage. Similarly, in medicine, beginner's mind liberates intuition; intuition can then inform my understanding, taking into account my prior ideas, successes, and failures yet remaining unfettered by them. Relying on expertise alone might produce a Dittersdorf,[8] but hardly a Bach; in medicine, it might produce someone who seems to have all the answers but doesn't ask the right questions.

A FLAG IN THE WIND

Gary, a friend of mine, was diagnosed with bladder cancer several years ago—the slow-growing curable kind, fortunately. He had cystoscopic surgery and was sent home with a catheter. After a few days, the catheter was removed, but he got into trouble—he had intense pain when he tried to urinate and developed urinary retention. The catheter was reinserted for a few days and then removed again— on a Thursday afternoon. On Friday, he started having abdominal pain that grew in intensity during the day. His urologist's office was closed, so he went to the busy emergency room of a well-respected California hospital. The physician noted that Gary had little urine output, so he started an IV, perhaps assuming that Gary was dehydrated. He signed out to another physician, who noted that Gary was still not urinating much, so he increased the rate of the IV. They continued the IV drip overnight. In distress, Gary's wife called me early the next morning. Gary was in agonizing pain. I spoke to the nurse on his unit, and I insisted that he be seen by the urology resident. Before the resident arrived, though, the nurse checked Gary's abdomen and said, "Oh my God, your bladder is about to burst." She placed a new catheter, draining two liters of urine from Gary's bladder. He eventually did get well, but he spent two additional days in the hospital before going home because he developed a fever due to a (preventable) kidney infection.

In one sense, this case defies the imagination—how could well-qualified doctors and nurses persist on an erroneous path when an alternative and logical explanation—recurrent urinary retention—would be perfectly obvious to someone with no medical training? It's a striking example of cognitive rigidity—the resistance to changing one's thinking or beliefs, a tenacious adherence to one view of reality. Every clinician can think of a time when he or she fell into a trap like this. In medicine, manifestations of illness are polysemous—they can be interpreted in many ways—creating a field of cognitive traps into which clinicians routinely fall. When harried, clinicians are more likely to stop thinking when they find the first, and not necessarily the best, of multiple interpretations of a situation. Cognitive scientists call this "search satisfaction."[9] Their interpretation then becomes ossified into a rigidly brittle—yet flimsy—"truth."

Novelist F. Scott Fitzgerald once said that "the test of a first-rate intelligence is the ability to hold two opposed ideas in mind at the same time and still retain the ability to function."[10] With the same contexts, scenes, and characters, one could write two completely different plays. Here, the doctors caring for Gary didn't consider the possibility of two different story lines—the dehydration story and urinary retention story. They settled on one of the two and considered it fact, even though the dehydration story was a poor fit. Having once committed to a viewpoint, clinicians can be extraordinarily unwilling to consider another, even if it is a better fit; changing one's mind is a source of shame, rather than a source of wonder. Gary's situation is even more remarkable because all indications suggested that the treatment was not producing the desired effect, even from the beginning—it would be odd for someone who was dehydrated not to urinate after two liters of extra fluid had been pumped into his system. The cognitive rigidity of one clinician was contagious, practically becoming a shared delusion among several health professionals. One definition of insanity is doing the same thing over and over and expecting different results.[11]

Part of the problem is the fast-paced environment of clinical medicine. Clinicians feel under pressure to come to a diagnosis and treatment plan and move on to the next patient. Part of that pressure is internal, though—something about the quick thinking is

exciting for physicians. Clinicians need some way of alerting themselves to the possibility that their understanding is provisional and
incomplete, that their expertise can lead them astray. They need a
trigger to help them slow down when they should.

The fast pace of medicine is only part of the problem. It takes
effort to hold two opposed ideas—to consider that a patient can
be *both* a great case *and* a suffering person, to see the relevance
of both the patient's experience and your own diagnostic formu-
lations. The ability to tolerate—and even embrace—ambiguity is
central to being a good diagnostician. Master clinicians see that
seemingly contradictory perspectives might offer explanations for
an evolving situation; they have the cognitive flexibility to let go of
ideas when those ideas are no longer useful. They can see how an
illness is caused by a virus *and* by the failure of the body's immune
system—and thus allow a wider range of treatment options. They
can see that a patient who doesn't take his diabetes medicine regu-
larly is both "noncompliant" and also "struggling to do the best he
can"—and that way the clinicians can mobilize support while also
encouraging the patient to do a better job. Mindful clinicians can
feel confident while retaining some doubt. Just the other day I had
to ask a colleague a simple question about a newborn (I don't have
many in my practice anymore). It was almost embarrassing, something any intern would know and I knew but needed to make sure
I had it right. It takes humility to recruit additional expertise.

A Zen story goes:

> Two monks were watching a flag flapping in the wind. One said to
> the other, "The flag is moving."
>
> The other replied, "The wind is moving."
>
> Huineng, their teacher, overheard this. He said, "Not the flag, not
> the wind; mind is moving."[12]

Seeing a situation from two perspectives simultaneously can reveal
an even more profound truth. Of course the flag is moving and the
wind is moving. What we don't always appreciate is how our minds
move between two or more views of the world. The ability to hold

contradictory perspectives is not only a marker of a great clinician, it also characterizes great scientists. Physicist Niels Bohr is reported to have said "the opposite of a fact is falsehood, but the opposite of one profound truth might very well be another profound truth." For him it was not intuitive to consider that light is both a wave and a particle—a paradox that boggles the imagination—yet the scientific evidence allowed no other explanation.

HOLDING EXPERTISE LIGHTLY

The failure of Gary's clinical team to adopt more than one perspective may have had its roots in an inability to adopt a stance of "not-knowing." Their expertise—or, better yet, the misapplication of their expertise—led to overcertainty, an arrogance in considering their provisional formulation to be an immutable fact. I can only speculate about what was going on in the minds of the clinical team at that time; haste and cognitive overload were likely at play, but there may have been more.

Not-knowing is not the same as laziness. In Suzuki Roshi's words, "Not-knowing doesn't mean that you don't know." Not-knowing means not letting what you know get in the way. It means "to hold what you know lightly, so that you're ready for it to be different."[13] In this way, knowing and not-knowing are not incompatible; they are two sides of the same coin.

Living each moment recognizing that our understanding is incomplete—maintaining a sense of "unfinishedness" in the fast-paced, information-overloaded world of clinical medicine—is not easy. Once I make a diagnosis, I notice that I tend to see information in a different way; anything that conflicts with that sense of "truth" makes me uncomfortable, even more so if I've made a commitment by having declared that truth to someone else. It's dangerous when you feel that it's better to appear certain even if you're wrong than to appear in doubt.

The discomfort that happens when you are confronted by new information that conflicts with your existing beliefs, ideas, values, or behavior—"cognitive dissonance"—is amplified when your sense of certainty is disrupted.[14] Faced with cognitive dissonance, we tend to seek consistency to lessen that sense of disruption. Traditionally, psychologists have identified two primary ways we relieve cognitive dissonance—by changing our ideas, values, beliefs, or behavior to accommodate the new information, or by plowing ahead, favoring information that confirms the old ideas and ignoring or rationalizing that which does not.[15] Too often, we shape the facts to conform to our beliefs. In medicine, patients' accounts of their illnesses are rich with inconsistencies, while chart notes are filled with seemingly coherent stories that confirm a diagnostic impression. Master clinicians find a third route, neither changing their viewpoint nor engaging in delusion. They practice living with the paradox. They accept that there might be two equally legitimate ways of viewing a situation, at least for the moment. Sometimes this paradox can be resolved as the situation evolves and new information becomes available. Other times, clinicians need to learn to live with uncertainties that might never be resolved.

In medicine, up to a third of the symptoms that patients bring to their doctors defy our attempts at diagnosis, and despite doing all the right exams and tests, we aren't able to provide a coherent explanation for the patient's distress.[16] Primary care physicians see scores of patients with leg swelling, which can sometimes be a sign of a life-threatening condition—a blood clot or heart failure—but most often is harmless. More than a third of patients whom cardiologists see with chest pain are found not to have heart disease. Neurologists' offices are filled with patients who are dizzy, but extensive testing reveals no clear diagnosis. In those cases, good clinicians hold on to a sense of unfinishedness for months or years. They know that the next time the same patient reports a symptom, it may prove serious. Clinicians, however, are prone to divide patients into those with serious disease and those with "functional" distress. Some illnesses defy Western medical diagnostic categories and appear to be mind-body illnesses. However, classifying those forms of distress as "functional" can also be a trap; clinicians can miss seemingly similar symptoms that represent something more serious. For example, a patient of mine had chronic unexplained abdominal pain for years. She had undergone extensive diagnostic testing, and no treatments helped. Her pain worsened when she was depressed. I saw her on a Friday and reassured her that it was likely the same pain that she had had for years, even though she protested that the pain was different that day. Three days later she saw one of my partners, who sent her for an ultrasound. She had gallstones. I had completely missed the boat. After surgery, *that* pain resolved. But she still had the same unexplained chronic pain. She had pain that was both unexplained and explainable. This paradox—a patient with two similar symptoms—is common. After a heart attack, patients commonly have aftershocks—chest pains that prove innocuous. Patients with rheumatoid arthritis often have fibromyalgia, too—muscular aches and pains that are not associated with any joint destruction.

DARING TO COME UP EMPTY

Zen is rich with stories that contain evocative pearls of wisdom. One of those pearls is about emptiness. As Suzuki Roshi explains, "If your mind is empty, it is ready for anything." The idea of emptiness is a radical, and somewhat disturbing, notion. One popular Zen story tells of a professor who once visited a Japanese Zen master to inquire about Zen.

> The master served tea while the professor expounded about philosophy. When the visitor's cup was full, the master kept pouring. Tea spilled out of the cup and all over the table.
>
> "The cup is overflowing!" said the professor. "No more will go in!"
>
> "Like this cup," said the master, "you are full of your own opinions and speculations. How can I show you Zen unless you first empty your cup?"[17]

On one level, this Zen story—and the concept of emptiness—is about making space so that we are ready for new ideas and can use our limited cognitive capacity more effectively.[18] The educator and philosopher John Dewey captured this spirit in the early twentieth century. Dewey called for emptying the mind as "a kind of intellectual disrobing." He said, "We cannot permanently divest ourselves of [our] intellectual habits. . . . But intelligent furthering of culture demands that we take some of them off, that we inspect them critically to see what they are made of and what wearing them does to us. We cannot achieve recovery of primitive naïveté. But there is attainable a cultivated naïveté of eye, ear and thought."[19]

As recently as thirty years ago, some psychologists believed that the message in this Zen story was nonsense. They believed that we had no risk of the cup's overflowing because we only used a small part of our brains in everyday life and that the capacity of the brain was nearly limitless. This idea—that we only use 10 percent of our brains—has achieved urban-legend status and continues to be stated as fact in the media and pop-psychology publications. Despite its appeal, the 10 percent idea has been proved wrong; research has repeatedly demonstrated that we use all parts of the brain, and that the brain has limited capacity for attention, memory, and problem solving. Doctors, like other high-functioning professionals, need all of their cognitive capabilities—and then some—to deal with the complexity of patient care.

The brain is prepared for overload, however. Your brain is always employing mental shortcuts; you categorize, summarize, see similarities, and aggregate information. That way, you achieve mental economy and process more information more quickly. But mental efficiency comes at a price; by characterizing a patient with a certain set of symptoms as an "example of X," doctors can miss a patient's unique features. As I'll discuss further in the chapter on decision making, efficiency can result in superficial solutions to complex problems.

Emptiness is more profound than simply making space in an overcrowded brain. Emptiness is a way of understanding the world. While objects in the world are real, emptiness means that the theories, categories, and labels that we apply to them are constructions of the mind (or collectives of minds) and therefore lack substance. This idea comes from the Buddhist philosophy of emptiness (as I mentioned in chapter 1) and was also articulated by William James, the father of American psychology and a self-described "pragmatist."[20] James held that mental categories—such as diagnoses—can seem so real, but are fundamentally fragile. They have explanatory power but must be set aside in favor of other ways of seeing the world when their usefulness is tenuous and unproven. Expertise means knowing when to dare to come up empty.

By now it should be clear that assigning a diagnosis can both illuminate and obscure clinicians' thinking. A patient of mine was first considered a "classic" case of temporal lobe epilepsy, then, of borderline personality disorder, bipolar II disorder, post-traumatic stress disorder, and somatization disorder. Ironically, each of these explained her distress, but each was fundamentally unsatisfactory—the patient was all of these and none of them. This flux is true in all areas of medicine. Despite years of evidence that the underlying cause of stomach ulcer is a bacterial infection, doctors were reluctant to give up their notion that stomach ulcers were due to poor nutrition, stress, or excess acid production. Similarly, doctors took years to follow evidence-based guidelines to use beta-blockers to treat heart failure. Until the 1990s, we were all taught the lore that beta-blockers would weaken the heart, not strengthen it. It took over a decade for the medical profession to fully assimilate a new worldview.

Doctors are trained to cling to categories. In medical school one of my professors said that there were 10,000 diseases. That was in 1984. In 2015, the *International Classification of Diseases* (*ICD-10*) listed over 170,000 different diagnosis codes. In medical school, students learn about "cases" of a particular illness before learning how to care for people who are ill. We learned to call diseases "diagnostic entities," as if diagnoses were "things" that exist in the world, like a table or a kidney. You confuse the living, breathing human being in front of you with the diagnosis codes in a chart.

TWO KINDS OF INTELLIGENCE

There are two kinds of intelligence: one acquired,
as a child in school memorizes facts and concepts

from books and from what the teacher says,
collecting information from the traditional sciences
as well as from the new sciences.

With such intelligence you rise in the world.
You get ranked ahead or behind others
in regard to your competence in retaining
information. You stroll with this intelligence
in and out of fields of knowledge, getting always more
marks on your preserving tablets.

There is another kind of tablet,
one already completed and preserved inside you.
A spring overflowing its springbox. A freshness
in the center of the chest. This other intelligence
does not turn yellow or stagnate. It's fluid,
and it doesn't move from outside to inside
through the conduits of plumbing-learning.

This second knowing is a fountainhead
from within you, moving out.
                    —Jellaludin Rumi (1207–1273)
                    translated by Coleman Barks

The poet Rumi provides a compelling description of beginner's mind. Rumi lived in thirteenth-century Persia, and his writings have enjoyed a well-deserved renaissance in the past few decades; his words are often amazingly timely. In an often-quoted poem,[21] Rumi describes the familiar analytic kind and another kind of intelligence—a "fluid" intelligence and a "freshness" that comes from within. This other intelligence is first-person knowing, the kind of knowledge that emerges from stories rather than textbooks, from reflection rather than analysis, from immediacy rather than categorizing. The "freshness" that Rumi summons is beginner's mind— avoiding being blinded by theories, facts, and concepts, and living a truth, not just describing it. Only eight hundred years later has cognitive science caught up with Rumi's prescience, and now medical educators and psychologists affirm that these two approaches are necessary for good clinical judgment, being complementary and not incompatible.[22]

Prior to the twentieth century, doctors commonly talked about diagnosing the *person*; only later did doctors talk about diagnosing *diseases*. In ancient Greece, and in traditional Chinese medicine, disease was seen as an ever-changing dynamic imbalance of humors.[23] I am not advocating abandoning modern medicine in favor of ancient practices (although some of these too may be effective). Rather, we can learn from those older traditions in the way that they recognize that people are dynamic, their symptoms and experiences change, and their illnesses have trajectories—making the case for clinicians to ask themselves, "Is there something new or different with this patient today?"

Unfortunately, diagnosing people in this dynamic way is not reinforced in current clinical practice. The force in medicine that drives billing is the codable diagnosis—sadly, a billing category. Until beginner's mind is supported by the structure of health care organizations—and I believe that it can be (more on this later)—it needs to come from within, no small task.

THE WATER JAR TEST

Those who engage in meditation have claimed that in doing so they can promote beginner's mind. The trick is in how to prove it. Psychologists had to find a way to observe and measure beginner's mind, or its opposite, the tendency of the mind to be "blinded by experience," known as the Einstellung effect—when rigid thought patterns get in the way of identifying more adaptive and creative solutions to a problem.

A team of Israeli researchers came up with a way to measure the Einstellung effect—the Einstellung water jar test.[24] Typically the water jar test is in two phases. In this experiment, volunteers were trained to solve several problems (dividing water in different ways among several jars of different sizes), each of which required the same complex formula. Then the volunteers were given a new problem, which could be solved using a much simpler approach, and were left to their own devices to figure it out. Those who had prior mindfulness practice figured out the simpler solution more readily. As a researcher, though, I wasn't convinced. For example, the same qualities that led someone to undertake meditation practice might also be the ones that led to better performance on the test.

The researchers then took people who had never done any contemplative practice, meditation, or attention training and divided them randomly into intervention and control groups. An eighteen-hour intervention program over seven weeks introduced five different practices—attention training (focusing on the breath), body scan, open awareness, walking meditation, and compassion meditation—plus various awareness exercises, dialogues, and home practice.[25] Those in the intervention group scored better on the test, less likely to be blinded by experience and more likely to find simpler and creative solutions. They had learned to adopt a beginner's mind.

IN THE CLINIC

Over the years I have developed a habit of pausing momentarily before entering any patient's room. With my hand on the doorknob, I quietly take a breath to help me become more present in preparation for the visit—I mentally set aside everything that has happened with the patient I have just finished seeing and other events of the day so that I can be fresh and available. I let go of expectations. It takes just a second or two and invites the freshness that Rumi describes.

I am not the only one to discover ways of achieving mindfulness-in-action. Julie Connelly, a physician colleague at the University of Virginia, writes eloquently about how poetry can promote beginner's mind.[26] Rumi's poem and other poems that invoke the same openness of mind are now on my computer's screen saver, a reminder to balance my view of each patient, to see through an analytic lens, bringing all of my knowledge, expertise, and experience, and also to cultivate a "freshness" within.

Reflective questions keep me on track and out of trouble. I habitually ask myself, "Is there another way to view this situation? What am I assuming that might not be true? How are prior experiences and expectations affecting how I view the situation? What would a trusted peer say?" These "opening-up" questions help me identify my cognitive rigidity and blind spots, some of which are the consequence of the expertise I worked so hard to develop. Reflective questions are not about factual recall; rather, they are questions that open up one's awareness, raise doubts, and expose uncertainty. Anyone who works in a complex environment (and who doesn't?) will find that questions such as these do lead to greater mindfulness. I use the same questions with students and colleagues. Although I rarely talk about it in this way to students, reflective questions promote what the educator Donald Schön called reflection-in-action;[27] they take little time — a few seconds here and there — and save time in the long run. It's a way of remembering that while I might be good at finding answers, it's more important to know that I'm asking the right questions.

5

Being Present

I delivered babies for many years as part of my family practice. At first, I found it difficult to look directly at the face of women experiencing the intensity of labor. Reflexively, I'd avert my gaze. Witnessing raw and unfiltered expressions of pain made me feel uncomfortable and inadequate. I'd busy myself with a task—check the electronic fetal monitor, talk to the patient's partner, talk to the nurse. When I was doing something—prescribing a medication, actually helping a newborn glide into the world—I felt calm and confident. But I foundered when the situation didn't demand action—or demanded inaction. Perhaps patients noticed, or perhaps they didn't.

I undertook a practice of presence. I began, consciously, taking in each patient's face, recognizing yet resisting the urge to look away. I became aware of my own gaze and my facial expressions, noting when I drew back. I discovered that observing is not necessarily seeing. I could observe a woman's labor without seeing the person. Observing is much like what the philosopher Michel Foucault called the "clinical gaze"—a way of viewing a patient as a disease, a diagnosis, a clinical problem, somewhat less than a person.[1] In contrast, by not merely observing, and instead *seeing*, I could explore what it was like for me to be present.

Gradually I grew more comfortable. Distance—physical distance and emotional distance—seemed to dissolve. I no longer felt that I was going to drown. I could be more helpful, seeing ways in which I could relieve patients' discomfort. It felt genuine, intimate.

At first, presence was an interior experience for me; only later did I realize that it was shared. Patients responded differently when I was present. They looked back, they took my hand. The presence I could bring to a woman in labor seemed like the presence I felt as a performing musician. Being present had an impact on the care I delivered. I discovered what good midwives always knew—that you can "tell" when a woman is progressing in labor; this "telling" depends on presence. I was better able to wait before acting.

THE INEFFABLE

At its most basic, presence is made visible when the clinician makes good eye contact, responds to patients' concerns, and doesn't stand up and leave before the conversation is finished. However, when patients say their doctor is "really there," most patients are referring to a quality of being. Presence is a sense of coherence and imperturbability. Internist Tony Suchman calls it the "connexional" dimension of care, often unspoken.[2] Presence is a quality of listening—without interrupting, interpreting, judging, or minimizing. In case you hadn't noticed, doctors don't do this well. When psychologist Kim Marvel and I analyzed audio-recorded primary care office visits, we saw how doctors would get restless and take control after patients had spoken for an average of only twenty-three seconds.[3]

The philosopher Ralph Harper, in his book *On Presence*,[4] considers presence to be a "bonded resonance" in which two people are in touch and in tune with each other. Presence, according to Harper, is especially important in "boundary situations," times when people feel vulnerable, when life is particularly uncertain and when it's hard to find meaning. In medicine, these are times when patients face serious illness and loss of function, when patients and their loved ones are frightened, when there are unexpected mishaps. Presence is a gift of dignity and respect when patients need it most. Harper also points out that presence is always shared with a real or imagined other; presence requires a witness, even if that witness is another part of oneself—an observing self.[5] In that way I can be present with a patient even when a patient is unable to speak for herself.

I feel a bit daunted in trying to characterize presence, to render the ineffable visible and leave it no less wondrous. Presence has historically been the domain of poets, philosophers, and mystics; however, it is at the core of health care. When clinicians write about presence, they rarely do so using clinical language. They write stories.[6] Surgeons, internists, family physicians, and psychiatrists have described how you cannot force presence into existence, nor does presence reliably happen on its own; you have to make space within which presence can emerge. In that sense, presence depends on emptiness, getting yourself out of the way, setting aside inner chatter—what the Buddha called "monkey mind"—to connect more directly with a person, a task, or a part of yourself. Societally, more than ever we crave presence with ourselves and shared presence with others, patients and clinicians included. With our attention increasingly parsed among tasks that compete for the same set of neural pathways, we are divided into too many fragments—too many to maintain a sense of being whole. Every day our sense of presence is constantly being fractured and repaired—an exhausting prospect. Try having a conversation—a meaningful conversation—while entering data on a computer. At the least, your sentence structure becomes disjointed and you lose your train of thought.

PRESENTNESS OF TIME

Sometimes a simple gesture and a few well-placed words can signal presence. One day on rounds in the hospital, as we walked into the room, Laura Hogan, a nurse-practitioner on our palliative care team, said three words to the patient: "What beautiful flowers." The patient looked at the flowers and smiled. The previous day the patient had had a biopsy that would let her know whether her cancer had progressed; she was still awaiting the results. We all feared that the news would not be good. Laura's comment communicated that even in dire circumstances it is possible to see beauty and to honor those who loved and cared for the patient, that she was not alone. More often, though, presence is communicated nonverbally—a softness of gaze, a quality of touch, a handshake that is felt genuine rather than perfunctory, a gentle examination of a patient's tender abdomen.

Presence is also "presentness" of time. When I feel that I'm being present while caring for patients, time seems to expand or stand still. Several years ago, I went to a jazz concert by Chick Corea's group. During the opening piece, after each of the musicians had had a chance to improvise, the music reached a resting point, a silence that probably only lasted two seconds. Even though the concert was in a three-thousand-seat auditorium, everyone seemed to feel the same sense of intimacy and connection in that silence. That moment had an exquisite spaciousness, as if the outside world had ceased to exist, a spaciousness that resolved only when the musicians simultaneously struck a chord marking a new section of the music. Think of speeches by Martin Luther King Jr. or Mahatma Gandhi. You are captivated, entranced, transported, and time seems to stop or ceases altogether.

When physicians are being present, patients feel that spaciousness. I remember the first time I felt it as a patient. I was in my late teens and had not been feeling well for over a month; I was weak, tired, and feverish, with a sore throat, headaches, and no energy. I would get better for a while, then it would come back. I had recently graduated from my pediatrician to a new "adult" doctor, whom I did not know well. He was thorough and gentle as he examined my ears, throat, neck, chest, and abdomen. I presume that the physical examination was normal and uninformative; it confirmed a diagnosis that he had already made.

Time seemed to stand still. I was worried; he was imperturbably calm. He was much older than I, but that didn't seem to matter; he was warm and his eyes had a softness. I felt that he understood me and my situation, and the distance between us seemed to dissolve. He said that he'd seen this cluster of symptoms, which was probably a lingering virus, and that time would heal. He ordered a blood test just to make sure. That's all I needed.

This was the first time I felt understood and cared for—honored and respected—by a physician. I carried his presence with me after I went home and found his virtual presence quietly reassuring; I was not worrying alone. A couple of weeks later, I began to feel more myself. His image came to me years later as I was contemplating going to medical school and later during the dark moments when I wondered whether memorizing names of bacteria and reciting differential diagnoses was all that it could be about.

Later still, I discovered that I could be present in that way—and share my presence with patients. I had a new patient in my practice—Haqim, sixteen years old, muscular, confident, and robust. He had acne on his back and shoulders. He asked question after question—about hormones and how they affect the skin (and why they make people unattractive), how each medication worked, whether he could try two of them at the same time, and how long it would take for the bumps and cysts to go away.

He was worried—very worried. I listened, without interpreting or reflecting—I just listened. I explained that time would heal, with the help of a few creams and pills. After a few more questions about how the pills actually worked, he relaxed and even smiled. We spent the remaining five minutes of the fifteen-minute visit talking about his family. Since then Haqim has mentioned to me on more than one occasion that he wants to become a doctor.[7]

TIME AND INTIMACY

How can presence happen, though, when office visits are constrained to a mere fifteen to twenty minutes or even shorter? Elapsed time might be out of a doctor's control to some degree, but perceived time can always be created. I teach physicians to sit down while talking with a patient, rather than standing; in a study of surgeons making quick hospital rounds, patients felt that doctors actually spent more time when they sat down, even though the elapsed time was the same as when they stood.[8] A research colleague, Kathy Zoppi, found that parents were more satisfied when they *perceived* that pediatricians spent more time with them—the true elapsed time didn't matter as much.[9] Sometimes time is created through silence. As in music, where silences can have the same exquisite beauty as notes, silence can deepen a relationship between a doctor and a patient. It doesn't take much—a few seconds at most—to reassure a patient that the doctor is there, listening, attending, not rushed.[10] Using silence effectively is even more relevant now that visits—in the hospital and in office practice—are crammed with more administrative imperatives.

Musicians know about presence and its absence. When you're caught up in your thoughts and just going through the motions, your professional colleagues will say you're "just phoning it in." And you'll think, "I played a good concert. Wish I had been there." It's the same in medicine. When you're being present (or when you're phoning it in), patients know and you know. My mentor George Engel would say that patients want to know and understand and to feel known and understood. There's a difference between merely knowing *about* a patient and *knowing* the patient as a person. *Knowing* is much more personal and intimate. During training, supervisors and colleagues warned me of the dangers of becoming too involved with patients. Patients die, and they are ravaged by unspeakable tragedy, depredation, and abuse. Getting too close to the edge of this vortex feels dangerous. You fear that you'll lose perspective and degenerate into a mass of emotional jelly. Clearly, though, boundary situations require a *greater* sense of presence— not less. Only with a radically tenacious shared presence can a clinician maintain the sense of intimacy necessary to truly be there with a suffering patient.[11] In medicine, trainees hear little about how to do this. Staying coldly objective seems safer. It also has its perils. While doctors sometimes have to distance themselves emotionally as a survival strategy, making detachment a habit sterilizes clinical care of its richness and meaning. For me, being present means aiming for the sweet spot in which I am emotionally accessible to myself and others in a way that clarifies my vision of the patient, his clinical situation, and our relationship.

Dirk is a seventy-year-old man with paranoid schizophrenia

whom I have had in my primary care practice for over twenty years. Dirk has spent nearly all of his adult life in mental hospitals and group homes. He'd usually be laconic during our visits: I'd ask questions and he'd answer in a word or two. Over the past year, Dirk has had several episodes of passing out or nearly passing out. His blood pressure was low, likely a side effect of his psychiatric medications. While none of his injuries were serious, I was worried. That day, Dirk was his usual emotionally flat self; I couldn't tell what he was thinking. He recounted having fallen in a stairwell with the same monotone he'd use if he were reading a list of telephone numbers.

Then I said, "I'm worried," and waited. To my surprise, Dirk became more talkative. He said that he was worried too. We talked about the risks and benefits of lowering his medication doses—which might help with the episodes of passing out, but might risk worsening his psychiatric condition. He then talked about how it felt to be different, the stigma of his mental illness. I was speechless; I had completely underestimated his insight.

This brief exchange opened up a new chapter in our long relationship. In the past, I didn't feel that we had achieved any kind of connection. It took twenty years for that moment to emerge, and I now see him as more of a whole person. It's reciprocal—I get the sense that now he sees me as a person, not just "the doctor." Periodically I wonder if I had never given him a chance, that by doing the habitual doctorly things—asking questions, poking, prodding, giving advice—I had inadvertently silenced him. Now we, together, had the opportunity to make a better decision—to lower his medications. I am better able to advocate for him and to address his housing and medication needs and the social activities that give his otherwise impoverished life meaning. Dirk has slowly become more disclosing, sharing more of himself. I have a better understanding of what he fears, what he needs, what he enjoys—and who he is.

STORMY SEAS

Laura Kerner was seventy years old and enjoying her retirement until she had a heart attack followed by pneumonia, septicemia (infection in her bloodstream), and a blood clot to her lungs. During her four weeks in the hospital, despite intensive treatment, she was declining; her heart did not have sufficient reserve; she was suffocating for lack of oxygen; her liver and kidneys were failing; she was dying. She had previously said that she would not want life support if she was not expected to survive.

As the days passed, Laura had fewer and fewer lucid moments and was increasingly agitated and delirious. Suctioning her oral secretions would provoke coughing spells. Drawing blood required multiple attempts. Even moving her in bed made her short of breath and she had to be restrained to keep her from pulling out her IVs. Distressingly, the ICU team had to withhold painkillers and sedatives because they tended to lower her blood pressure. As her chances of a meaningful recovery diminished, her physicians and nurses grew increasingly distressed.

As a palliative care consultant, my job was to help Laura, her family, and the ICU team make important decisions about her care, but no one could agree on anything. Some family members thought Laura would want hospice care, whereas others demanded that "everything" be done, "no matter what." Each day the family divisions grew more acrimonious. Her son would say, "You doctors are trying to kill my mother," "You're just giving up," "She's always been a fighter and you're taking that away from her."

Doing things—explaining, offering opinions, directing—had already backfired; I certainly was *not* going to tell them what to do. All I could do was be attentive and present. I found it easy enough to be aware of my feelings of irritation and anger and my judgments about her family's motives (Are they uncaring?), capacity (Are they paranoid? Do they really understand?), and morals (Are they irresponsible?). It was another thing to set those feelings aside and welcome their questions and take in each of their views. I'd have to consider the possibility that I misperceived their motives and see my own contributions to this mess—perhaps by having taken sides when I shouldn't have. I had to cultivate a sense of hospitality.

THE GUEST HOUSE

This being human is a guest house.
Every morning a new arrival.

A joy, a depression, a meanness,
some momentary awareness comes
as an unexpected visitor.

Welcome and entertain them all!
Even if they are a crowd of sorrows,
who violently sweep your house
empty of its furniture,
still, treat each guest honorably.
He may be clearing you out
for some new delight.

The dark thought, the shame, the malice,
meet them at the door laughing and invite them in.

Be grateful for whatever comes,
because each has been sent
as a guide from beyond.
                    —Jellaludin Rumi
                    translated by Coleman Barks

The presence I was seeking had been described in a poem, "The Guest House,"[12] in which the poet Rumi commands you to welcome into awareness the dark thoughts and feelings of chaos, disruption, and powerlessness, and to respond deliberately—by being available, open, receptive, and—yes—cheerful. Easier said than done, I thought. I tried slowing down. I would take a breath and wait before responding—to make sure that I was not reacting out of anger or impatience and was not severing the tenuous connection I had with them. I invited *them* to slow down too. Even with the pressures to rush to a decision, I encouraged them to take a few more minutes to make sure they were comfortable. Eventually, they seemed more present too. They could finally respond thoughtfully to the question "Right now, what are the two or three things you'd most wish for— for Laura and your family?" With the passing days, they allowed us to provide pain medications and attend to Laura's comfort under their close watch, and they could not but notice that she was more peaceful, more comfortable. To my amazement, after she had died a few days later, her family expressed gratitude for our team's care.

MAKING SPACE

Cognitive neuroscientists are now beginning to consider how the interior and personal experience of presence manifests in the brain. As you can imagine, studying presence is one of the hard problems of neuroscience—much harder than studying attention, memory, or perception—because it is so subjective. In exploring the meager research on presence, I was surprised with what I found. My sleuthing led me to research on video games and virtual reality, environments in which people become so fully immersed that they feel that the situations are real, sometimes even more real than real life. Players enter into relationships with humanoid avatars, experiencing a sense of shared presence as if their "companion" were alive. The electronic medium and all of its artificiality seemingly vanish, and people achieve what the Italian neuroscientist Giuseppe Riva calls "embodied immersion";[13] your sense of self dissolves, perhaps like the feeling of presence that musicians, teachers, and doctors feel when they're at the top of their game.

In case you're thinking that video games are mindless and far removed from clinical practice, think again. They aren't. Computer programs now use avatars as virtual doctors and even psychotherapists—quite effectively.[14] Patients become emotionally attached to the computer figure in the same way that they might connect with a psychotherapist. Like Harry Harlow's monkeys, who, in captivity, bonded to an inanimate "mother" made of wire and cloth, humans naturally bond with other people, or what they imagine to be people, even when they know that they're not real. It's because our brains are wired to promote attachment and relationship.[15]

Social presence—or shared presence—is critical for health care. The ability of doctors to see each patient as a complete human being (and vice versa), in my view, is the basis for the trust and understanding that help the patient through the hard times. It is a learned skill, a habit of mind. It reminds me of how I'd prepare for concerts. Performing well in the rehearsal room was only part of it. I'd get the technique down and would let the music speak. Yet, I'd need additional practice to prepare for when I'd be onstage, in relationship with people who I imagined might be approving or critical, being moved or watching my every move. Similarly, clinicians have to prepare for those relationships that place them outside their comfort zone—when there is suffering, conflict, uncertainty, or loss.

It might seem straightforward how humans come to be present with and understand one another. After all, we have language and can communicate what is important to us. Yet shared presence goes beyond language. Philosophers and cognitive scientists have explored how we come to understand the minds and intentions of others, even though it's hard enough to read our own minds, much less those of other people. They emphasize that, as social beings, we *need* to understand others' internal experiences in order to cooperate, collaborate, communicate—and survive. Until recently, human understanding was thought to involve "theory of mind," that we constantly theorize about what might be going on in others' minds—what they're aware of and what they're thinking and feeling. Sometimes we try to verify whether our "theory of mind" is correct; but more often we do not. Those who lacked theory of mind were particularly impaired, such as patients with autism and schizophrenia.

A competing theory about how we understand each other is called embodied simulation, which proposes that we relive in our own bodies and minds the actions and presumed intentions of the other. For example, when I used to do deliveries, I would find myself holding my breath and straining when women were experiencing contractions; I would do this without being aware of it, then it would filter into my consciousness. I entered the raw sensuality of the experience (albeit vicariously). At the same time I could also be aware of my "doctorly" frame of reference; I'd say to myself, "When you're holding your breath and straining, perhaps it's because you know that the patient is entering the second stage of labor."

More recently, social neuroscientists, psychologists, and philosophers have taken another step further. Theory of mind and embodied simulation suggest that we are separate entities, that it is one mind understanding the completely distinct mind of another. This is only partially true. Research suggests that our minds are intertwined, so much so that it seems that our minds are not completely our own. Some part of our cognitive and emotional lives—and our identities—is shared with others.[16] I am not merely an aloof observer of a patient's experience; I am, to some extent, a participant. In that way, presence is intersubjective; it blurs the boundaries between that which is *me* and that which is *you*.[17] Intuitively this makes sense. We engage in shared mental processes all the time; married couples commonly complete each other's sentences, and doctors and patients might both recognize in the same moment that something is wrong.[18] The premise of the field of "team science"—how teams work together—is that teams have shared mental models.[19] Science has only begun to describe how shared mind happens, psychologically and neurobiologically, and the implications are profound.[20] I believe that we are at the cusp of understanding how presence happens—when shared mind is revealed to both parties.[21]

LIKE ME, NOT LIKE ME

Presence—unfortunately—is not naturally democratic. Humans are not only social organisms, we are also tribal—for better and for worse. We connect more easily with people we perceive to be similar to ourselves. "Tribe" can be whatever we define it to be—the tribe of white people, the tribe of those who speak Portuguese, the tribe of the sick, or the tribe of the poor. You might consider yourself a member of several tribes at once. As a result of their—often unconscious—tribal affiliation, people tend to see the world through a particular lens, consciously and unconsciously dividing the world into those whom they perceive as being "like me" and others who are "not like me."

Physicians are tribal too. Perhaps that's why doctors are poorly prepared to be patients when they themselves become ill. When physicians become ill, they really don't like it. Doctors don't only feel more vulnerable because of what they know (. . . and now they're going to do *that* to *me*?), they literally become strangers to themselves.[22] It's as if doctors and patients belong to different tribes, and when doctors become ill, they become involuntary members of both.

While the positive side of tribalism is a sense of belonging and communion, the dark side is bias—a set of unverified and preconceived assumptions about someone, often simply because we think that they belong to a particular group. Everyone harbors biases, whether it be about race, ethnicity, gender, body habitus, sexual behaviors, or something else.[23] Physicians, like everyone else, make different assumptions about people depending on whether they are obese or thin, male or female, black or white, Spanish-speaking or English-speaking, and a myriad of clinically relevant and clinically irrelevant factors. These biases usually are implicit—below the level of awareness.

These biases affect the care that patients receive.[24] When physicians' tribal associations prevail, the seeds of bias are sewn. Witness the early days of the AIDS epidemic, when people who superficially were very much like their treating physicians—well educated, predominantly white, generally healthy males—were "othered"; they were blamed for their illness and sometimes treated as if they were less than human. Staff left hospital food trays at their door, afraid to enter the room. Physicians avoided touching them—even long after everyone knew that HIV was only spread through intimate contact and blood products. They were made into outcasts, in part driven by clinicians' fears—of stigmatization by association, of contagion, of talking about sexual and drug use behavior, and of death.[25] While now—fortunately—the horror stories about clinicians' refusal to care for patients who were HIV infected are well behind us in most communities in the United States, this dynamic persists in large parts of the world.

Tribalism is hardwired in particular parts of the brain—the dorsomedial prefrontal cortex in particular—which respond differently if we feel that the other person is a member of our tribe. Tribalism is expressed through our hormones. Oxytocin, the hormone that promotes labor and milk production, also promotes love and nurturance within one's tribe. However, for those outside one's tribe, oxytocin has the opposite effect—it promotes aggression (think of why it's not a good idea to get between a mother bear and her cub).[26] In case you were wondering, men have oxytocin too, with the same psychological effects. Our tribal tendencies are to some extent a survival strategy—evolutionarily, we've always needed to be able to assess quickly who was friend and who was foe.[27]

The discovery of mirror neurons in the 1990s revolutionized neuroscience by providing a mechanism for human understanding. Mirror neurons fire when we observe others engaging in goal-directed tasks such as reaching for an object (the early experiments used monkeys witnessing other monkeys reaching for food). These nerve cells are located near our motor cortex—the part of the brain that controls our movements—and when they are activated, our brains simulate what it is like for the other person (or monkey) to engage in that action and thus draw conclusions about the other's intentions and goals. More recently, scientists have speculated that some areas of the brain interpret not only the physical actions of others but also their associated emotions. These emotional resonance systems are thought to be the basis of emotional intelligence and social intelligence. One such area—the anterior cingulate— seems to grow and develop in response to mindfulness training.[28]

Being present with a patient (or anyone for that matter) whom I perceive as "not like me" initially feels less natural than with others with whom I share aspects of my identity. I will admit that—initially—I relate more effortlessly to a fellow professional than to someone who is mentally ill or to a recent refugee from an embattled third-world country. It takes effort and imagination to resonate with the other person's experience. I have to ask, "What's it like?"—and hearing the answer usually connects me with a more basic and shared human experience. My brain needs to shift gears to bridge the gap between my life and his.[29]

A PRACTICE OF STILLNESS

Practicing presence, for me, is practicing becoming available (to myself and others) and practicing quieting the mind. Being available means showing up and letting patients know—through words and gestures—that there is space. Patients can recognize presence when they don't feel that they have to say, "I know you are busy, but . . ." or "Sorry to bother you with . . ." Clinicians are afraid of being too available—myself included. They're afraid that patients will call them at all hours of the day and night and invade their personal lives relentlessly. Even though I know that's a real risk, I have to remind myself that being more available often saves time. At the end of a visit, I'll say that usually I'd schedule a follow-up visit in a month, but that they can come back sooner; they usually say no but appreciate knowing that space is there. Sometimes I give out my home phone number to patients who are worried or are seriously ill. Patients rarely call, and in thirty years of practice, I can count on one hand the patients who called inappropriately. Knowing that they can reach me makes them feel that I'm present. I find that they call the practice less often; they don't feel a need to repeat and amplify their concerns.

Quieting the mind makes space within the clinician; it promotes openness. For those who are drawn to it, sitting practice offers one way to quiet the mind, and the presence that is achieved while alone can translate into presence with others. Among doctors who take the time for stillness, nearly all feel that the time one makes for contemplative practices—meditation, reflection, awareness—is soon recaptured in increased clarity. The goal of presence is not necessarily efficiency, but efficiency often arises from presence.

All contemplative practices offer ways of practicing stillness. Yet these practices do not confer immunity to strong emotion; quite the opposite. Even those who've spent thousands of hours meditating have the same kinds of reactions to stress as anyone else.[30] Their hearts race, they feel anxiety and dread, and they experience moral outrage. Research shows that these immediate emotional reactions are at least as robust in experienced practitioners as in those who've never done any contemplative practice. So why bother? The difference is that in experienced practitioners, those stress reactions abate sooner—they don't keep on reverberating. Rather, experienced practitioners discern more rapidly which emotions and experiences are "theirs," and which belong to other people—in other words, they're good at self-other differentiation.[31] They have the skill to "decenter"—they can feel their own emotions and at the same time observe them as if they were standing outside themselves. They develop a capacity for what psychologists call mentalization—they understand their own mental states rather than being oblivious of or mystified by why they feel the way they do. They have learned to see their mental states as something they can control rather than the other way around; they know that these states are transitory and not enduring, that they ebb and flow. For example, they more readily distinguish between *I am* feeling *angry*—an emotion that they can control—and *I am angry*—a person whose anger is part of their identity. They learn to set aside their immediate reactions so that they can respond more mindfully.[32] All of these skills open up space for presence. Physiologically, meditators learn to regulate the expression of certain genes that affect the number and type of receptors to the stress hormones (such as epinephrine, cortisol) that course through our systems when we're aroused and anxious, as well as the neurotransmitters (such as serotonin, dopamine, neuropeptide Y) that play a role in regulating emotion.[33] It's not that you don't have strong and sometimes-distressing feelings; while feeling their immediacy, you learn how not to be consumed or paralyzed by them.[34]

WHERE ARE MY FEET?

You can practice presence. One way is a practice called "Where are my feet?" At first glance, it seems almost too simple. Ask yourself, "Where are my feet?" Give yourself a moment to feel your feet. Are they flat on the floor? Is your weight equally on both feet? Is there any discomfort? Do you feel them inside your shoes? Do they feel strong and reliable? Pay attention to any sensations you might experience. You can do this while standing or sitting. Once you get the hang of it, see if you can ask "Where are my feet?" in a stressful situation. Use it as a way to stay present. Feet are our foundations, our sources of stability, and our engines of mobility; they maintain balance, allow us to be still, and impel us forward. By assuming a physical attitude of stability, strength, and balance, you simultaneously draw attention to and stabilize your thoughts, feelings, and emotions.[35] Your physical presence stabilizes your presence of mind.[36]

Shared presence is cultivated through deep listening. In workshops, I frequently ask participants to write about meaningful experiences in their work settings, moments of connection and times when things did not go well. Participants pair off, and each is given time to read her story or tell it in her own words. However, this is not a social conversation; it's an exercise in listening deeply, with attention, curiosity, and beginner's mind. While it's okay to ask clarifying questions about what happened and how the other person felt, and also to express understanding or empathy when appropriate, I caution listeners to be aware of their impulses to interpret, criticize, judge, or elaborate upon their colleague's emerging story—and to deliberately set those thoughts aside for the moment so that they can be present. To help them respond more mindfully, I'll suggest that listeners have some way of slowing down. For example, if they feel that they have something brilliant or insightful to say, rather than saying it right away, they might count slowly from one to five, and only then share that insight if it still seems as urgent and relevant after the short wait. Deep listening can be remarkably difficult. It feels awkward. We're so used to thinking about our responses before the other person has finished speaking—we feel we have to be doing something and not just be there. With practice, though, most people feel gratified when listening deeply, knowing that the other person feels heard and understood in a space of shared presence.

Yet another way of practicing shared presence was described by Chade-Meng Tan, who created the Search Inside Yourself "mindfulness for engineers" program at Google. In a deceptively simple exercise that he calls Just Like Me,[37] you visualize somebody in your mind and then consider—and even gently speak to yourself—phrases such as "This person has a body and a mind, just like me. This person has feelings, emotions, and thoughts, just like me. This person has, at some point in his or her life, been sad, disappointed, angry, hurt, or confused, just like me. This person has, in his or her life, experienced physical and emotional pain and suffering, just like me. This person wishes to be free from pain and suffering, just like me. This person wishes to be happy, just like me," and so on. You can easily carry this contemplative practice with you into the workplace with colleagues; it's particularly useful with people with whom you don't see eye to eye.

With this and other practices of presence, you open the door to dialogue and understanding, and you build the mental muscles to prepare for the moments when you feel the least prepared. Practicing presence helps clinicians slow down, listen more deeply, think more deliberately, shift from doing to being and from activity to stillness. Practicing presence, even for a moment, can be long enough to avoid a potential error, long enough for a patient to feel acknowledged, heard, and known.

6

Navigating Without a Map

Richard Grayson was a retired professor of epidemiology. He had been a patient of mine for the previous ten years, and I was one of his sole supports during a messy divorce. He was a lover of good food and wine and now had no appetite and couldn't tolerate alcohol. He looked gaunt and tired. He had lost twenty pounds, his skin color was a pasty white, and his eyes were slightly jaundiced. I ordered a CT scan of his abdomen, knowing that the news would not be good. He had a stage IV cancer in his liver—which likely originated in his bile ducts—aggressive and incurable.

Richard wanted to know the facts. The cancer surgeon advised him that surgery would be risky and unlikely to improve survival or quality of life. Richard said that he would never consider chemotherapy, but I encouraged him to see an oncologist, just to find out. This muddied the waters. Richard learned that chemotherapy offered a 20 percent chance of extending his life by an average of a few months while possibly improving his energy and appetite. No one could know whether he would be one of the lucky ones whose cancer would respond—or one of the 80 percent who just had side effects with no benefits at all. He consulted another oncologist, searched the Internet, and wrote to friends and colleagues, including some of the most highly regarded oncologists in the world. The options were dizzying, including a "promising" experimental treatment. Richard knew well that only 5 to 10 percent of experimental cancer drugs prove effective, and no one knew what the side effects might be.

During his entire career Richard had taught students how to design and interpret the results of clinical trials and assess the risks and benefits of treatments. He understood the statistics of his own situation well and knew how his situation was different: the average patients in those research studies were younger and their cancers were less advanced. You couldn't imagine a patient who was better informed. However, the more information and statistics that Richard acquired, the more anxious and bewildered he became. His knowledge of medicine, statistics, research methodology, and probabilities carried him just so far. Despite being well-informed, he felt lost.

Now the decision—which had seemed easy before he started his journey—was harder. He kept changing his mind. He was frightened. A rationalist, he felt that his logical, analytical brain was being hijacked by emotions. Like most patients facing a serious and complex situation, Richard was experiencing cognitive overload; the stakes were high and emotions were raw, medical evidence was unclear, and the risks and the benefits weren't completely known. He came back to see me to help sort this out. He asked, "What would you do if you were me?"

Before I move on to what happened, sit with me for a minute. Imagine you're the physician in the exam room and this question was lobbed into your court. I knew that nothing was going to save Richard's life, that having to make decisions was adding to his burden, and that he was frightened and his fear made it hard for him to think clearly. Whoever made the decision, Richard would have to live with the consequences.

Physicians dread when patients ask, "What would you do if you were me?" As a physician, you're *not* the patient, but the patient wants you to be there, with him, helping him decide. In oncology, physicians have seen countless patients refuse chemo, then with the terror of death looming, change their minds. Thus it's understandable how a doctor might say, "I've not been in that situation"— technically true, but emotionally harsh. When the question comes from a patient who has a terminal illness, it's even more difficult because it brings the physician closer to contemplating her own death. Physicians too get anxious as their patients get sicker; doctors tend to avoid direct discussions of death in favor of focusing on scans, tests, and treatments.[1]

In a previous era when physicians comfortably assumed a paternalist role, the doctor's job was to assemble the facts and provide a plan: "We should start chemotherapy this Friday. My assistant can set it up for you." The patient's voice was secondary. Now things are a bit different, but things haven't changed *that* much. Patients are commonly offered a role in decision making, but doctors often make an offer that is hard to refuse, a choiceless choice. They might say, "Research suggests that for metastatic bile-duct cancer, chemotherapy with gemcitabine plus cisplatin offers the best chance of longer survival; it can give you more time—and in most cases it's high-quality time. And if that doesn't work for you, we have other options. Does that sound reasonable? If so, we can start this Friday." Some physicians will try to build the patient's confidence: "I've had two patients recently who did well on gemcitabine plus cisplatin in similar circumstances." Some offer numerous options and provide exquisite detail about the clinical research upon which their recommendations are based. Giving a nod to patient autonomy, a physician might say, "Go home and discuss the options with your family and let me know what you'd like to do," and if pressed, might even say, "I can't really tell you what to do. Everybody's different. The choice is up to you." But the patient hears, "Chemo or die."

Richard didn't need to know more about risks and benefits for people in general; he needed wisdom in *his* unique set of circumstances. He felt adrift at sea without a compass, navigating without a map. Few people want to make such decisions alone, if for no other reason than it's difficult to think through an issue logically and analytically when faced with our own mortality. Richard needed his physician not only to advise but also to help him understand his values and feelings, cope with uncertainty, sort out his options, and navigate his way.

I sometimes hear physicians say, "It's up to you." This allows them to remain aloof and displaces fear and uncertainty to the patient, leaving the clinician with a false sense of having been patient centered. Rather than promoting the intimate discussions that patients deserve in such circumstances, it disempowers patients by depriving them of the support that they need. They're abandoned to their rights.[2] No one wants a physician who is going to fall apart when facing the possibility of the death of one of his patients, nor do they want a physician who is Teflon coated, unmoved by suffering. Shared decision making is not only providing information; it is facing uncertainty together. That's why it can be emotionally wrenching for physicians too. They have to work with the anxiety that they feel when facing uncertainty, enter into the unknown *with* the patient. Eric Larson calls it "emotional labor"—the emotional work that is part of the job.[3]

In these circumstances, patients want to have their voices heard; however, they exercise their voices less commonly than you might think. I can imagine several reasons why. Having greater choice means assuming a greater burden of responsibility. They're overwhelmed by the sheer quantity of information. They may want to please the physician. Even well-informed, highly educated patients fear that by questioning their physician, they will get lower-quality care.[4]

These factors were weighing on me as I examined Richard's abdomen. I needed time to think. I did a careful exam, not expecting to find anything new, but the exam served two other purposes. I knew that touch, in these circumstances, communicates solidarity. It also allowed me time to regroup, to think about what I could say next, something that would move him toward a decision that was right for him. I sat for a moment with the "What would you do . . . ?" question. I did not want to diminish his question by merely providing an opinion. I assumed that he was looking for understanding as well as clarity and wisdom, not just information.

I said, "Let's walk through this." I started with larger questions, hoping that within them lay the answer to the more specific question about treatment choices: "What's the hardest part? How will you know that the choice is the right one? What in your life, right now, brings you joy? Where do you want to be living, and with whom? When will you know you've done enough? Is there anything about this decision for which you'd not be able to forgive yourself?"

After each question I was silent. Not trying to direct the conversation, I was just listening. The silences were just a few seconds each, but they had a quality of spaciousness, lending a deeper emotional tone to this discussion than the discourse of scans, tests, and drugs that had dominated most of Richard's prior visits with his physicians. Some of the questions went unanswered. It was hard to be silent; it would have been easier to dispense information, recommendations, reassurances. But, by choosing to live with the questions rather than fill the space with mere answers, something else happened. Those five minutes led us to a greater sense of shared understanding. My just listening exposed me to his angst, not just his dilemma. I understood him better and he understood himself better.

"I'm willing to take the chance with the high-dose chemo," he said. "But, I first need to ask whether I can switch to the low dose if it's too much for me." This decision was not "my" decision nor was it Richard's; it was shared, having emerged through conversation, through being together; the decision was navigation more than negotiation. I was surprised; I had misjudged him. Somehow I thought he—as a scientist—would have decided otherwise, given the actuarial odds. He wanted the moon shot and was willing to tolerate the pain.

While this may have been the right choice for *him*, others would have chosen differently. He had enough information and advice, so I asked and didn't recommend. Richard had few side effects from the chemo and enjoyed a reasonable quality of life until six months later, when the tumor again started to grow. He was soon in hospice; he felt that he had made the best choices under the circumstances; he had no regrets.

IT DEPENDS

Health planners Sholom Glouberman and Brenda Zimmerman describe decisions as simple, complicated, or complex.[5] Richard's decision was hardly simple, but Mary Ann's was. A twenty-five-year-old software engineer with all of the typical symptoms of a urinary tract infection, she saw me the same day as Richard. She'd had a similar episode the previous year that resolved after a day of antibiotics. It didn't take much to come to a diagnosis and prescribe an appropriate treatment. The choice among two or three potentially effective antibiotics was based on cost and convenience. I simply followed a recipe, something that barely requires medical training.

But what if Mary Ann also had a high fever and back pain that suggested it was more than a bladder infection? Let's say she had diabetes or kidney stones. Or she was pregnant. This is more serious. The stakes are higher. The decision about which tests to order and which antibiotics to use and whether she needs to be hospitalized also depends on a myriad of social factors such as whether she has someone at home who could watch out for her and whether she has insurance coverage. This is now a complicated problem.

Glouberman and Zimmerman describe complicated problems as a bit like sending a rocket to the moon—you need more than a recipe. You need knowledge and formulas and the expertise to know how to consider a myriad of factors, from ambient temperature to wind speed to availability of personnel to guide the process. Still, the goal is clear and unwavering. There might be several possible trajectories, but all use the same principles of physics. Having sent a rocket to the moon once makes you more confident that you can do it again.

A typical complicated decision is the choice between lumpectomy (removing part of the breast) plus radiation, or a total mastectomy, for breast cancer. Although the treatments offer an equal chance for long-term survival, patients have to live with the trade-offs: convenience, quality of life, body image, and risks of recurrence. Each patient has to figure out what *she* wants, not what anybody else might want.[6] Doctors can help patients choose, recognizing that the patient's choice may differ from what they might want for themselves.[7]

Richard's problem was beyond complicated—it was complex. In

the words of economist Charles Lindblom, in the face of complexity people "muddle through."[8] They set an initial goal, then reorient and redirect their efforts based on evolving information. This is not necessarily a bad thing. Complexity means unpredictability and competing imperatives, and the goal may not be clear until having embarked on a path. At the outset of his illness Richard might have said—like most people—that he wanted to live longer, enjoy a good quality of life, maintain his dignity, and be with family and at home. Sometimes all goals are possible to achieve, but for people with serious illnesses, often they are not, and decisions—such as the decision to embark on chemotherapy—are provisional and conditional. If Richard had had a bad reaction to his first round of chemotherapy, it's likely that he'd have changed course.

Complex decisions have always been part of medical practice. But, in the past twenty-five years, complexity has skyrocketed. In 1990 there was one medication to treat AIDS; now there are more than twenty-five that can be combined in many ways. Ditto for cancer. For nearly every disease I treat as a family physician, including diabetes, heart failure, and high blood pressure, the options have expanded exponentially, and the guidelines that purport to simplify them are ever changing.

In the face of complexity, the mind strives for efficiency. Too often—to paraphrase H. L. Mencken—we find an answer that is "clear, simple, and wrong."[9] Being mindful, in contrast, means taking in the full catastrophe and being reluctant to oversimplify;[10] you use protocols and guidelines but aren't constrained by them; you don't indulge in an illusion of certainty when ambiguity prevails. You assign a diagnosis and continue to maintain an open mind. You know when to break rules and by how much. You know when to seek patient input that can lead to even better choices.

Part of what I love about my work—in family medicine and in palliative care—is that there is a map, but like the areas on navigational charts from the early explorers that blur into the background, it just doesn't have enough detail. In a cookbook that I picked up in India, one of the recipes instructs to add "asafetida to taste" and "cook until nice," not particularly helpful instructions if you've never cooked Indian food before. It feels that way in clinical practice sometimes. Even for common conditions, the answer often is "It depends . . ."[11] Working with complexity requires what William James called "a large acquaintance with particulars"—details of patients and their lives—"that often makes us wiser than the possession of abstract formulas, however deep."[12] The particulars I deal with every day have to do with knowing each patient as a person, his genetics and habits, how he responds to illness, whom he lives with and whom he cannot live without, and how his wishes and aspirations affect his decisions. Finding out what makes patients tick is detective work, the kind of work that anthropologists and investigative reporters do, a human science, recognizing that every patient is, to some degree, an "n-of-1 study," without a control group, and that you have to rely on intuitions and gut feelings. You need know how the patient's world and your own world intersect.

PRACTICAL WISDOM

In medicine, knowledge of diseases, diagnoses, guidelines, and clinical evidence carry you just so far. When you're choosing a doctor, you want one who has something that Aristotle called *phronesis,* loosely translated as "practical wisdom." *Phronesis* is about choosing which actions will serve *this* patient best, right now. William James said, "All human thinking is essentially of two kinds—reasoning on the one hand and narrative, descriptive, contemplative thinking on the other."[13] Good decision makers use both.

Wise decisions in the face of complexity require the whole mind—the thinking mind, the sensing mind, the feeling mind—not just the logical/analytic mind. Just as Richard needed to feel his way through a complex situation, I needed to feel my way too; logic was not enough and the decision was not merely an actuarial task. Nor was it discovery in the usual sense; we did not add to the facts of the case. The decision was relational. We collectively made sense of a bewildering set of information and, to do so, invited multiple perspectives—mine, his oncologists', his family's, his own; we asked questions, built stories about how different choices might devolve, and created partnerships that enabled Richard to clarify his values, goals, and preferences—to exercise his autonomy. This was an intimate project, not merely tolerating ambiguity but embracing it.[14]

SHARED MIND

In my visits with Richard we moved—sometimes haltingly, sometimes directly—toward something I've come to call shared mind.[15] Talking about a "mind" that was shared between us and yet is owned by neither of us is no longer the province of science fiction; as I described in chapter 5, shared mind is at the cutting edge of social neuroscience research. Social neuroscientists are now able to describe how two minds collaborate, how thoughts, emotions, and sensations are constantly shaped by the social relationships that surround us, so much so that thought is shared. "Hyperscanning" research—in which two individuals' brains are scanned while they consider a shared task and communicate with each other—shows how the same areas of the brain are activated in both people to an astounding degree.[16]

I find the neuroimaging research provocative because it sets the stage for interpersonal mindfulness. Just as *intra*personal mindfulness is about knowing one's own mind—one's intentions, aspirations, goals, and foibles—*inter*personal mindfulness is about knowing others'. In all human interactions, we read one another's minds—our intentions, emotions, and thoughts. Doctors do it and so do patients. Mind reading is tricky, though. We make inferences about others' thinking based not only on what we consciously see and hear, but also from information that is outside of everyday awareness; even the beginnings of a smile, a tone of voice, or a brief glance away can build or undermine a relationship (if you're in doubt, read Austen or Proust). People also "read" and respond to each other's pheromones—those smells that we give off that provide subliminal signals about attraction, anxiety, and anger.[17] Our olfactory neural pathways go directly from the nose to the emotion-sensing parts of our brains, in particular the amygdala, which likely also affects our moods and the decisions we make. In this soup of neurotransmitters, deciding together in the face of complexity and strong emotions requires more than one mind. Richard needed to recruit additional help to come to a decision. In this case, two minds were better than one.

A STIFF NECK

I was an intern working in the pediatric emergency department when a young child came in with a high fever in the middle of a frigid January night, brought by understandably worried parents. A respiratory virus was going around. I was hoping that was all it was. I examined the child—irritable, crying. I had been taught that "irritable and inconsolable" equals a hospital admission, and I was relieved when his mother consoled him after a few minutes.[18]

The child was warm to the touch and had a fever of 39.5°C (about 103°F). Protocol in these situations called for a careful physical examination focusing on finding an explanation for the fever, and if no explanation could be found, to do a lumbar puncture—a spinal tap. His eardrums were a bit red, likely from crying and not from infection, and he had a cough but no signs of pneumonia. The examination was otherwise unrevealing.

Then I examined the child's neck to assess if it was stiff or supple. He did not like being taken from his mother's arms, and as I flexed his neck gently, he cried and reached for her. I tried it again, with him in his mother's lap, and it went a bit better. His neck didn't feel stiff—or at least not stiff enough to be called "stiff." But it wasn't really supple either. I flexed his neck again, noting that he didn't flex his hips; if he had, that would have been a classic sign of meningitis. I was a bit relieved, but not completely so; still I needed to convince myself that the child would be okay. I drew some blood and sent it off to the lab. A few minutes later the results came back; the white count was normal, and that tipped the balance. I could now justify not obtaining spinal fluid. I sent the child home and told his parents to bring him back to the clinic in the morning, just a few hours hence.

I went back to the on-call room, but I didn't sleep well, a telling sign that something still felt unresolved. In retrospect I knew that I had convinced myself that things were more "all right" than they might have been. That this all happened at four in the morning changed everything. To do a lumbar puncture, I'd have needed to wake my supervising resident. He was somewhat disagreeable. He'd say that he didn't "mind" being woken at night, but I and others knew otherwise. So I didn't wake him. Had it been at four in the afternoon rather than four in the morning, I would likely have done the lumbar puncture. Fortunately, within a few hours the child had improved. But not doing the lumbar puncture simply because I didn't want to face the possibility of humiliation was still the wrong choice. This time I was lucky, and so was the child; another child with the exact same symptoms and lab tests could have had meningitis. A near miss. Next time I might not be so lucky.

To put all of this into perspective, I'm not alone. A recent article by oncologist Ranjana Srivastava chronicled how she didn't speak up about the safety of planned surgery for a lung tumor;[19] her gut told her to contact the surgeon, but she didn't because she assumed that the surgeon—who was well-known and well-respected—knew what he was doing. She was right and the surgeon was wrong; the patient died. Three other physicians later voiced that they had had doubts, but were afraid that they might have been wrong and so didn't speak up. The surgeon was horrified that others perceived him to be so intimidating.

It is not just in the emergency room, in cancer surgery, or in terminal illness that complex decisions arise. In primary care, I often have to assess which patients with uncontrolled type 2 diabetes should start insulin injections rather than continue with their oral medications. On the surface this might seem a simple problem—there *are* clinical practice guidelines about this issue. However, the real wisdom of clinical practice is to know when to break the rules. In the past couple of years I've broken the diabetes rule several times—with an obese man who was successfully losing weight and whose diabetes would likely improve if he continued, with a woman with progressing metastatic breast cancer, with a homeless young man with a history of suicide attempts who had panic attacks at the thought of a needle, with a frail eighty-year-old woman who wouldn't live long enough to suffer the long-term consequences of diabetes, with a woman who lived alone in a remote location making it harder to get help if she had an insulin reaction. Each of these situations required *phronesis* based on an appreciation of the particulars; amassing more facts and calculating probabilities would amount to what internist Faith Fitzgerald called "the punctilious quantification of the amorphous,"[20] trying to divide a raw egg by slicing it with a sharp knife. No matter how sharp the knife, you end up with a runny mess. The knife is a good tool, just not the right one.

Nonetheless, physicians are now judged by that punctilious quantification. If I don't prescribe insulin and the patient's blood sugar becomes slightly out of control, my care will be considered inadequate even if tighter control might actually have made the patient's health worse;[21] the patient is now considered to have "uncontrolled diabetes," the medical assistants in my office flag the chart for special attention, and insurers consider it a blemish that justifies denying financial bonuses based on "quality."

Glouberman and Zimmerman point out that addressing complex problems is like raising a child. The goal is a healthy outcome, not necessarily a predictable or identical one. If you have more than one child, each turns out differently, even if you've provided the same love, nurturance, guidance, caring, and patience. If you're fortunate, each child will live a fulfilling life, but in different and unpredictable ways. Parenting books and advice are helpful but only up to a point. Then you have to muddle through. As soon as you feel a sense of mastery, though, a new phase arises for which you are again unprepared. There is no clear path and sometimes no map at all.

DECISION SCIENCE

In medicine, sometime in the 1960s decision making was elevated from the realm of intuition and experience to what is now called decision science. By the 1970s, experts proposed that medical decisions be made based on clinical evidence.[22] Clinical questions would be translated quantitatively, such as "Consider a hundred patients with atrial fibrillation [an abnormal heart rhythm that can lead to blood clots and strokes]. Assuming that their risk of stroke is about 5 percent per year, how many patients would you have to treat with blood thinners to reduce the risk of stroke to 2 percent?" No one wants to have a stroke, but blood thinners have their downsides too—not only hemorrhage, but also the annoyance of getting blood tests every week or two to adjust the dose of the medication. It's a balance. To address the balance, researchers developed the concept of "utilities" to quantify the degree to which a life with a small stroke would be worth living, and the degree to which taking a blood thinner, going for frequent blood draws, and the possibility of a hemorrhage would diminish quality of life. This approach often displayed decision trees with multiple branches, each branch ultimately leading to the "right" decision in a specific circumstance, depending on the individual's level of risk.

Proponents of decision algorithms were puzzled when the algorithms were infrequently adopted. They learned that clinicians and patients just didn't think that way, nor did they *want* to. The idea that every patient would have the same "utilities" seemed particularly presumptuous; individual patients might have different values and preferences than the group as a whole,[23] and modeling the sometimes-unstable preferences of individuals faced with complex decisions quickly becomes a statistical nightmare. These models tended to assume that humans are rational decision makers, a proposition that is both attractive and ludicrous—attractive because it improves the likelihood that decisions reflect our underlying values, and ludicrous because so many nonrational factors influence the choices that we make. Psychologists Daniel Kahneman and Amos

Tversky, for example, described how decisions framed as avoiding a loss result in different choices when framed as opportunities for gain.[24] Their experiments explored how humans are not entirely rational even when they seem to be acting logically, and that the biases and heuristics that drive decisions are often below the level of awareness. If a close friend had a complication from a particular medication, wouldn't you feel a bit more reluctant to take it—even if you knew that complication was a one-in-a-million event? And if you were that friend's physician, wouldn't you also be more reluctant to prescribe it even knowing that the chance of the same event happening twice is vanishingly small? Recognizing that patients and physicians are just as vulnerable to unconscious biases as anyone else, decision scientists embraced models of "bounded rationality."[25] But if we're not entirely rational and biases are below the level of awareness, how do we monitor them? Here's where metacognition comes in—literally thinking about your own thinking (and feelings too), regulating your inner operating system, or, in emergency-room physician Patrick Croskerry's words, regulating your own "mindware."[26]

As Croskerry points out, good decisions require a kind of education that most clinicians don't yet receive—an education about how their own minds work so that they can more readily assess their biases and engage strategies to correct them. This "education" is more than reading a book about neuropsychology. He adds that de-biasing involves uncoupling one's observations from expectations, interpretations, and premature judgments. Good decisions also require mental stability, affect regulation, and clarity of purpose—in a word, mindfulness.

Research now demonstrates how attention training and compassion training can increase awareness of our own biases and thus reduce their influence on decision making.[27] Through training, implicit mental processes—including biases—are more accessible to awareness. You hesitate for a moment before reacting; you become more discerning and you uncouple expectations (what you think you'll see) from observations (what you do see). You reconsider.

INTUITION

In medical school we were taught a protocol for diagnosing skin conditions. We'd describe the location of the lesions, their color, whether their margins were distinct or fuzzy, whether their surface was smooth or scaly, and whether they were raised or flat. Based on those features we were taught to propose a list of possible diagnoses, rank them in order of likelihood, and select the most likely. This seems simple enough, but it's not the way that experienced dermatologists actually diagnose skin lesions. When experienced dermatologists try to follow the medical student protocol, they fall down; instead they rely on first impressions.[28] Similarly, experienced doctors know when a patient's story just doesn't "add up" or something doesn't quite "look right."

At first, decision scientists tried to debunk intuition. This is understandable. They were trying to correct the excesses of a prior generation of physicians who, in their arrogance, believed that the care they delivered was better than their colleagues' and relied only on anecdotes to support their views. In their zeal, though, decision scientists were blind to the opposite problem, that when decision making is totally dominated by analytic thinking, doctors get into a different kind of trouble. The challenge is to cultivate an informed intuition that can guide but not completely dominate the decision-making process.

Intuition is murky, visceral, impressionistic, and irrational, making it difficult to describe and study. However, intuition is vital for making sense of complex situations. The current generation of decision scientists take intuition seriously, but still have difficulty describing what it is and how it works. That is because, in part, intuition isn't just one thing, and it goes by different names—gut feelings, fast thinking, fuzzy traces, Type 1 processing—each of which is slightly different in its emphasis on thoughts, emotions, visceral sensations, and memories.[29] Some types of intuition may be employed when encountering familiar problems, such as the dermatologists' pattern recognition, whereas other types of intuition act as a guide to novel situations by helping the decision maker see similarity or analogy to prior situations, or they involve emotional or social intelligence—how to know and interact with others.

In the last decades of the twentieth century, groundbreaking work by neurologist Antonio Damasio suggested that the ability to make wise choices depends on awareness of one's own emotions and those of others—a view that had previously been considered radical by research psychologists and cognitive scientists. In his book, *Descartes' Error*, Damasio discusses the case of Phineas Gage, an unfortunate man who, in 1848, sustained a severe brain injury that impaired one of his frontal cortices, the part of the brain that confers awareness and regulates emotions. Mr. Gage survived the injury, and the rest of his brain was remarkably intact. His memory and abstract logic were good and he could carry on normal conversations. He was able to hold a job, at least for a while. Yet, according to his physician at the time, Gage's personality changed; he was "manifesting but little deference for his fellows, impatient of restraint or advice when it conflicts with his desires, at times pertinaciously obstinate, yet capricious and vacillating, devising many plans of future operations, which are no sooner arranged than they are abandoned in turn for others appearing more feasible."[30] With the loss of his prefrontal cortex, he had lost the ability to recognize and regulate his emotions, anticipate the consequences of his actions, or learn from his mistakes; as a result many of his personal decisions were disastrous.

It makes sense that emotions and intuitions would be important in making life choices. Imagine if this weren't so. Few people would choose a life partner by starting with a list of attributes, then going down a checklist with each potential candidate until the one with the most points wins. Most of us would consider the potential partner's list of attributes while also listening with the heart and the gut—messages from the body that only later can we frame as part of the story of falling in love. This may be as true with complex medical decisions; clinical evidence can only take us so far, and the heart and the gut must also speak.[31]

If emotions, social cognition, and intuition are essential to decision making, how can they be cultivated? The clinician who is will-ing to engage in the inner work that it requires has two main tasks: moving from fragmented mind to whole mind, and from individ-ual mind to shared mind. Evidence suggests that the potential for whole mind and shared mind is innate. But physicians' professional training undernourishes these capacities.

SAYING NO

A colleague, Stu Farber, died of acute myelogenous leukemia at age sixty-seven. Stu was a palliative care physician and was dealt a diffi-cult and rare diagnosis, one from which only a quarter of patients live for five years and even fewer are cured. In an article written shortly before his death,[32] Stu recounts that he was hospitalized with pneu-monia. The chemotherapy had predictably suppressed his immune system. The infectious disease consultant explained that while Stu's pneumonia was likely due to a virus and would likely resolve on its own, it might be a more lethal infection, Pneumocystis, the agent responsible for most of the early deaths from AIDS. To tell the dif-ference between a virus and Pneumocystis would require an inva-sive lung biopsy under sedation, but given how ill Stu was, there was a greater risk of complications from the procedure, and at best it would take him a few days to recover.

Stu knew that he was dying, but if this was Pneumocystis his life might be prolonged with treatment. His doctors implied that not to do the procedure would be unthinkable, but the pulmonologist still asked, "What do you want to do?" Stu was caught between two worlds—his familiar world as a clinician and the new, and strange, world of being a patient. Fortunately, Stu had the presence of mind to say that he was now comfortable and didn't want to rock the boat; he didn't want the biopsy and would take his chances. To his surprise, the physician then said, "That's the same choice that I would make."

What is stunning about this story and many others like it is that physicians can make very different choices when it comes to their own care than what they might recommend to their patients.[33] Physicians tend to recommend the most aggressive care for their patients, even when that care is likely to cause further discomfort and disability. Yet, when physicians themselves (reluctantly) join the "tribe of the sick," they may want fewer aggressive life-prolonging measures, instead focusing to a greater degree on their comfort and dignity.

How could this be? Even in his final weeks of life, Stu was astute, seeing that while his physicians couldn't easily place themselves in his shoes, they might be able to move beyond protocol and cold logic and appreciate the patient's perspective. But it took prompting by a particularly clear-sighted and knowledgeable patient. Here, Stu's physician, like many others, breathed a sigh of relief when Stu chose to forgo aggressive treatment and to focus on comfort—it unburdened the physician from having to make the decision. But few patients have the knowledge and the clarity to question physicians' recommendations and would benefit from physicians' efforts to apply a beginner's mind to decisions that initially seem self-evident.

BEING A DOCTOR BEING A PATIENT

As I was recovering from an attack of kidney stones, my primary care physician ordered an ultrasound of my kidneys to determine if there were any residual stones. I had had stones before, and a number of ultrasounds and CT scan reports were in my medical records. The ultrasonographer was friendly and chatty, and I enjoyed being able to make out a few anatomical structures on the screen as she scanned my left kidney (where the stone had been), then my right. She seemed to be taking a particularly long time on the right side and taking a lot of snapshots on the computer. Then she went quiet. I noticed that she was lingering quite a bit north of kidneys, ureters, and bladder; we were in liver territory. Perhaps she had found a gallstone, I thought.

I asked what was going on. Generally, technicians are not supposed to reveal findings until they are confirmed by the attending radiologist, but she knew that I was a doctor and had also been looking at the screen. She was reticent at first, then said, "There's something interesting I need to check out with the radiologist." In medicalese, *interesting* is never good. The radiologist explained, "Not only had the ultrasonographer looked at the urinary tract, she also noticed something going on in the liver." She had found an incidentaloma—a baseball-size something-or-other that apparently no one had seen before. I had no interest in having it be *my* incidentaloma; it was an unwelcome guest.

Over the past twenty years I have become personally acquainted with several incidentalomas. In medical slang, an incidentaloma is a surprise, a mass or lesion unexpectedly identified during a routine examination or imaging procedure—X-ray, scan, or ultrasound—or during surgery. Originally referring to benign tumors of the adrenal glands that were completely harmless, the term is now applied to any mass that you're not looking for. Incidentalomas make simple situations complex. While an incidentaloma is usually of no clinical significance, it isn't always. Occasionally, it might be cancer.

The radiologist was diligent. He went back to a CT scan from seven years before, also done after a kidney stone. There it was. No one had noticed it because they weren't looking for it; they had no reason to look for a liver mass. Even with my untrained eye, I could see a subtle shadow there. The radiologist estimated that in the seven years since the CT scan, it had grown in diameter by one millimeter. He was sure that it had grown; the scans are quite accurate. He thought it looked like benign nodular hyperplasia, a harmless nondisease that had gone undetected until scanners got more sophisticated and ultrasonographers more proficient. I did some quick calculations. One millimeter does not sound like a lot, but it might be a 10 percent increase in volume or even more depending on whether it was round or irregularly shaped. That's still pretty slow. I was fifty-two at the time, and I calculated that at that rate of doubling, I'd still have at least some of my liver uninvaded at age ninety. This did not provide much solace, though.

The options were to do nothing and take my chances, do a biopsy to get a definitive diagnosis and risk bleeding or infection, or do a series of MRI scans to see if it was growing at a detectable rate. But, at one millimeter every seven years, you'd have to do a lot of scans over a long time—expensive, unpleasant, and anxiety provoking.

A large part of my professional life consists of helping people make difficult decisions, and I thought of myself as quite capable of making difficult decisions in general. Or so I thought until I found myself asking the same question of my primary care physician that Richard Grayson had asked me only a few months previously: "What would you do?" Now I understood what it felt like to have all of the facts yet to be unable to decide—and how different it was to be on the other side of the stethoscope. My rational mind and emotional mind were at war. Rationally, I knew that one-third of the population has some kind of incidentaloma if you look hard enough, and that over 90 percent of these are benign—and that mine had all of the characteristics of a benign tumor. But it didn't help to hear about other people's incidentalomas because mine was *mine*. I was living with uncertainty—and it was different from anyone else's.

Having a good imagination was a curse. I was convinced that I had the worst kind of liver cancer. I just wanted it cut out, whatever it might be. I thought about whether I'd prefer to have a liver transplant in Rochester, or in Pittsburgh or in Cleveland, where they had more experience. Then I thought about canceling my appointment with my primary care physician, just wanting to forget about it entirely.

Fortunately, my doctor was a good listener. He didn't challenge my fears; he listened patiently. He was quiet for a while, then asked me what I was thinking. I said that I wanted to forget about it. He said he was anxious too and had consulted a couple of his colleagues, who also doubted that forgetting about it would be the wisest choice. That was not what I wanted to hear. I didn't like the idea of getting a biopsy. Nor did he. We chose a middle way—getting a scan every four months for a year. I didn't like that option either; it would prolong uncertainty for months, and even though I knew that the likelihood of finding something serious was small, I would be anxious prior to each test. Yet, I found solace in the knowing that the decision—and the anxiety—was shared. Just like Richard Grayson, I sought shared mind, not just advice or facts.

That I'm sitting here writing about my incidentaloma eight years later means that it is unlikely to be a cancer. But that doesn't mean zero. I chuckled when a few weeks later the MRI scan report identified yet another incidentaloma in my liver, most likely a small tangle of blood vessels, as well as a not-completely-simple cyst (as it was once described to me) in my right kidney that had been seen on a previous set of scans. The next two scans showed no growth of the liver mass nor of any of its "friends." My uninvited guests had become permanent cohabitants, ones with whom I had to make peace.

7

Responding to Suffering

The word *suffering* is strikingly absent in conversations among physicians and patients.[1] Physicians commonly talk about pain, disability, stress, coping, and quality of life. In the research world I inhabit, my scientist colleagues talk about diminished "health-related quality of life" and fewer "quality-adjusted life years." But none of these terms have quite the same meaning as *suffering*, which implies a more personal and pervasive distress, one that affects someone's identity—the ability to be oneself and to be in the world. Suffering is more than symptom checklists and "rate your pain from one to ten."

It's not that doctors don't know what it means to suffer; many people decide to go into medicine as a result of their own suffering or that of a close family member or friend. That suffering might not be dramatic or life threatening, but it usually does raise the specter of impermanence. For me it was childhood asthma. I wanted to understand what was happening to me, why I couldn't run more than a few yards without getting short of breath, why I was different from other kids, and what the future might hold. If I had been born a few decades later, I'd have explored everything about asthma I could find on the Internet. Instead, I turned to our home encyclopedia and learned all I could about asthma and, later, the human body and the illnesses that could afflict it.

But not until two years after college did I decide to change my life course from aspiring musician to physician. I was living in Amsterdam, studying music, and had taken a month off to visit a good friend who was on a Fulbright grant in Varanasi, the spiritual capital of Hinduism, on the banks of the Ganges. Here suffering was made visible. Amid the heat, noise, squalor, and wandering cows, I saw beggars with missing limbs, old men blinded by trachoma with spines deformed by tuberculosis, children with unrepaired cleft palates, and families that had never known anything but hunger. Occasionally, a black sedan with tinted windows would dodge the human and animal masses, carrying the materially content from one island of tranquility to another.

After a few days in Varanasi, I borrowed a bicycle and rode eight miles to the deer park in Sarnath, where the Buddha delivered his first discourse on suffering. By the end of the ride I was hot, dusty, and thirsty. And there, at the entrance to the deer park was an orange-juice vendor, squeezing oranges. The juice was delicious—so cold and sweet.

By the next morning I had developed a fever and abdominal pain. I felt bloated and weak and didn't want to move. I *saw* the vendor squeezing the juice, just juice, no water. Or so I thought. I later learned that orange-juice vendors were notorious for surreptitiously cutting the juice with (presumably contaminated) water. Typhoid was endemic.

I had to get tested. A bicycle rickshaw transported me to the clinic a mile away. There, in the waiting areas, I saw hundreds of people crowded into oppressively hot small spaces, spilling over into the street, wailing in misery and grief, with open fractures. Smells of blood, urine, and vomit. I was overwhelmed by it all and petrified about my own situation—I knew that people could die from typhoid.

A nurse quickly ushered me into a small room. The doctor was dressed in an immaculate starched white tunic. He took my symptoms seriously and examined me carefully. He said that I did not need to be hospitalized, but that I should have blood tests and return the next morning. The test for typhoid was negative, and over the next few days I recovered. But the images of suffering remained indelible. Only later did the irony of the situation—a visit to Sarnath and a lesson in suffering—dawn on me.

A few weeks later, back in Amsterdam, I was awakened before dawn by a viselike pain on the right side of my abdomen, extending to my flank and back. I suspected that it might be a kidney stone; I'd had a friend who'd had one and described it as the worst pain imaginable. His description was no exaggeration; no matter which way I moved, I couldn't get comfortable. Even more than in India, I felt desperate. I needed the pain to stop. Immediately. Again, I was scared.

Luckily, my roommate had a car. She drove me to the university hospital. The emergency room was quiet. I don't recall seeing other patients, even in the waiting room. Soon I was on a gurney, being wheeled down empty corridors, all painted stark white, no windows. The doctor too was all in white—white jacket, white pants. He told me that I'd need an X-ray. Then everyone disappeared and I was left alone in that sterile landscape, without a person in sight, squirming, writhing in pain, not sure what would happen next. One of the nurses came out from behind a closed door and told me to stop moving and not to moan. Then *she* disappeared. Minutes passed. Everything took on a surreal quality. Eventually, someone started an IV and someone else did an X-ray to look for the stone. With some IV pain medications I was pain-free within an hour or two. I went home and was even well enough to go to a concert that evening. In that respect, the care I'd received was excellent. One could say that my health situation had resolved itself.

Except it hadn't. I still felt shaken and vulnerable. And since the X-ray hadn't identified a stone, I was also left with uncertainty. With no definitive diagnosis, I went back for three follow-up visits. Each time, I was asked to produce a small specimen of urine, then interrupt the flow so the doctor could perform a vigorous rectal examination (the technical term, *prostatic massage*, doesn't fully capture the experience), then I'd produce a second specimen, again interrupting the flow, then I'd produce a third. I had two more appointments during which these urinary acrobatics were repeated, and I finally got up the courage to ask, "Why are you doing this?" The doctor explained matter-of-factly that because I had recently been in India, and because they had not identified a stone, they needed to test for other things, including tuberculosis. One clue, he said, could come from a culture of prostatic fluid. The prospect of TB did not sound good. If he had explained this in the first place, it would have left me feeling less embarrassed and also less anxious about what was going on. The TB tests were negative, and we all assumed that this was indeed a kidney stone. I was discharged from the clinic; the doctor's parting words were that I didn't need to come back and that I should drink lots of water. Since then I've had several more episodes. Now, I dread ending up in an emergency room where I might be mistaken for a "drug seeker" and denied pain relievers. Interestingly, no physician has ever thought to ask how having had kidney stones has affected me.

These illness experiences tipped the balance and pushed my decision to go into medicine. I resolved never to let any patient of mine feel abandoned in this way. I learned, in a visceral way, that doctors could reduce or worsen a patient's suffering not only through treatments but also by how they behaved and how they chose to share information—or not. I envisioned my job as not merely to prescribe treatments, but also to heal through sharing information, being present, and being kind. I had no idea how difficult that could be.

INCONVENIENT TRUTHS ABOUT SUFFERING

There are several inconvenient truths about suffering. The first is that even when diseases are considered "cured," suffering can persist. Recently, I cared for a young man who had worked as a skilled machinist. He had been cured of his leukemia with a bone marrow transplant. While this was clearly reason for celebration, he now lived in chronic pain from graft-versus-host disease, a condition in which the transplanted white blood cells—his body's new immune system—rejected the host cells from his own intestinal tract and skin. He could barely eat due to abdominal pain and nausea, and his skin was raw and prone to infection. At age thirty-five, he was facing amputation of both legs due to chronic, untreatable skin infections that had spread to the bone. He spent more than half of his time in hospitals and the rest recuperating at home, socially isolated and impoverished due to his illness. He could barely get out of bed, and his pain required high doses of narcotics. This situation was deeply poignant for his family and the clinical team; he was considered a "survivor," yet each medical "success" only seemed to increase his suffering. I noticed that clinical staff didn't relish entering his room—he was a living reminder of our failures.

Diseases that have no symptoms at all can also cause suffering. Recently I had a patient—also a physician—who was diagnosed with high blood pressure, commonly described as a "silent killer." At first he tried to convince himself—and me—that what he had was "white-coat hypertension"—when patients have normal blood pressure except when in the presence of a doctor. To make sure, I had him wear a blood-pressure monitor for twenty-four hours. I discussed the report with him a few days later, and even though there were only a few normal readings (mostly while he was asleep), he said to me, "I'm not really hypertensive; it's just that my blood pressure is high at times." I was surprised, because he—as a physician—would routinely prescribe antihypertensive medications to patients every day.

This physician-patient offered insight into why some people avoid coming to the doctor, and why others take their medications only when they feel "tense," or not at all. People feel differently about themselves when they are given a diagnosis; they go from being an ordinary citizen to being a reluctant patient. Sometimes they feel less well, or simply flawed, fragile, or not quite whole; sometimes, as studies show, they end up missing more days of work, even though the disease is asymptomatic.[2] I asked him why he was so reluctant to take medications. He said it made him feel like a failure. Having lived a life of healthy eating, meditation, and exercise, he thought that he could somehow manage to avoid high blood pressure despite a genetic predisposition, as if virtue could trump DNA. I said, "Genetics is powerful, isn't it?" We both wished that things might have been otherwise. The pills, which he ultimately was willing to take, might lower his blood pressure but not his sense of failure. About the latter, I wouldn't have known had I not asked.

Sociologist Arthur Frank recounts how he experienced intense health-related suffering even in the absence of pain, illness, or disease. A "suspicious spot" was found on an X-ray several years after a presumed cure of his testicular cancer.[3] He knew all too well that when testicular cancer recurs, often it cannot be cured. Contemplating harsh chemotherapy and an uncertain future, his anxiety was disabling. Ultimately, further testing proved negative—he was and is cancer-free—but he was struck by how his suffering during that waiting period went unnoticed and published an account as a reminder to physicians that "routine" diagnostic tests are rarely routine for the patient.

Even though doctors experience that same kind of anxiety as Frank when they themselves become patients, when in the physician role they find themselves glibly ordering diagnostic tests even for incurable illnesses such as HIV, lupus, or cancer. When executing the series of mouse clicks to order a test, I can forget that, at the same time, a patient might be contemplating his demise. Patients rarely speak up about this kind of suffering, perhaps assuming that it's not part of normal medical discourse. It takes just a moment to notice and acknowledge, "It's going to be a few days before we get the results, and I'll call when I know. How are you doing with all of this?"

THAT WHICH WE CANNOT NAME

The discourse on suffering went into hibernation during the years of impressive technological advances in medicine starting in the 1960s. I suspect that the heady optimism that accompanied the advances in our understanding of the mechanisms of disease and the promise of new treatments obscured the reality that these advances alone would not make suffering vanish. In fact, until the early 2000s, the tagline of the National Cancer Institute was an overly optimistic "to eliminate all death and suffering due to cancer by 2015."

Not until the 1980s was serious discussion about the nature of suffering and goals of medicine rekindled, by Eric Cassell, a New York City internist. Cassell was devoted to understanding communication between patients and physicians—when it worked and when it went awry. He remains a key figure in a countercurrent in medicine concerned with the human experience of illness.

Cassell first described suffering as a holistic experience where there is "severe distress associated with events that threaten the intactness of the person." This definition was radical. By looking at his own practice, as well as listening to and analyzing audio-recordings of consultations between patients and physicians, he realized that doctors often missed the point—they did not see patients' suffering. In a seminal article in the *New England Journal of Medicine* in 1982,[4] he reminded the medical community that the central obligation of healers is to address suffering—not just cure disease or relieve pain. He showed how suffering is only loosely associated with pain; that suffering itself has meaning, and that meaning can affect the severity and quality of a person's distress and the sense he makes of it. After all, the pain of childbirth can be more intense than that of a heart attack, but the overall experience is different—a joyous outcome rather than terror about the future.

Cassell showed how suffering is more than merely having a diseased part—a lung, a kidney, a brain; he said that suffering is experienced by whole persons. Other domains of suffering—psychological, existential, spiritual, financial, social—are often more devastating than physical symptoms. I've heard many chronically ill and dying patients say that the worst part of their situation is not the illness itself but the way the illness has impoverished or otherwise burdened their families. Cassell knew too that contact with the health care system can make a patient's suffering worse—"If we're not a part of the solution, we are a part of the problem."[5]

In the thirty years since Cassell's article, nursing researchers, medical ethicists, and those in hospice and palliative care have brought suffering out of the closet, especially for patients at the end of life. Still, it is remarkable how infrequently physicians ask about suffering. "How are we feeling today?" just doesn't get there.

Too often, doctors assume that they understand what is making a particular patient suffer most. The reality is that we usually do not.

In fact, physicians are cautioned *not* to use the word *suffering* for fear that it casts patients as victims, denying them agency and personhood. However, this can go too far. I once prepared a monograph for the National Cancer Institute on enhancing patient-physician communication. The subtitle was "Promoting Healing and Reducing Suffering." Though many of the scientists and clinicians around the table who were reviewing the monograph were supportive of the title and the approach, others were puzzled. They knew how to measure physical and mental health: physical, emotional, social, and existential quality of life; pain and other symptoms; and stress and coping. Nonetheless, healing and suffering were unfamiliar locations on their cancer map, even though most intuitively realized that suffering is not merely the presence of measurable pain or distress, just as health is not merely the absence of disease.

I recently reviewed the mission statements of thirty health care institutions around the country, many of which were impressively long and detailed. Not one mentioned suffering. Instead, they contained phrases such as "exceeding customer expectations," "eliminating cancer," "the highest order," "the best provider," and "trusted partner." One hospital's mission statement even suggested that physicians "treat the body," leaving the care of the hearts and minds of patients to others.

Next, I checked to see if the word *suffering* appeared in any of the 170,000 *International Classification of Diseases (ICD-10)* diagnosis codes that are used as the basis for billing, quality metrics, and health statistics. Not even once. Over the past months, I've systematically searched the medical literature for articles that explore how physicians can and should respond to suffering. I found a mere six research studies. Quite a number of thoughtful reflective essays provided compelling *descriptions* of suffering as well as physicians' and nurses' *attitudes* toward suffering; most addressed suffering in end-of-life care only; few touched on other contexts in which suffering occurs, and even fewer proposed ways of responding to it. Perhaps this is because suffering, being a holistic experience, doesn't neatly fit into the way that doctors and researchers tend to think. It is difficult to see—and address—that which we cannot name.[6]

SUFFERING BY ANY OTHER NAME

Karen Volk was in her late thirties when I first met her; she is now fifty-three. Karen was trained as a social worker and has two children. She had left an abusive relationship and was recently remarried. For years, she had been chronically fatigued, yet all her blood tests, including those for Lyme disease, anemia, lupus, thyroid disease, and a host of others, were normal. She complained of migrating joint pains and swelling, but a physical exam showed little of note. She had multiple tender points in her shoulders and back and did not sleep well, all characteristic of fibromyalgia—a poorly understood condition that is a minor annoyance for some and debilitating for others. She had also been diagnosed with interstitial cystitis, a painful bladder condition of unknown cause. For clinicians this is a familiar picture: chronic pain in multiple sites, fatigue, depression, and abuse tend to go together.[7] Her mood was like a roller coaster, but her symptoms didn't necessarily fluctuate with her state of mind or level of stress. A few years before, she had become dependent on narcotics for chronic pain; after having weaned herself off them, she didn't want to risk dependence in the future.

Every few weeks, Karen would land in my office, in pain. I prescribed medications for pain, depression, inflammation, and insomnia. Some were helpful, yet overall Karen declined, until three years later she could barely walk and could no longer work. The less mobile she became, the more weight she gained, putting on fifty pounds. And the pain persisted. At first, we tried to avoid narcotics, but nonnarcotic pain medications just didn't work for her. She had a high tolerance for narcotics and, despite the substantial doses that I prescribed, still had severe pain. The only option was to up her doses, which worried us both.

Before I met Karen, her chart had grown thick with consultations from infectious disease specialists, orthopedic surgeons, neurologists, sleep specialists, rheumatologists, dermatologists, urogyne-cologists, podiatrists, and mental health professionals. Rather than accept and work with uncertainty, some of her specialists created an illusion of knowing and control, proposing "functional" diagnoses—fibromyalgia, migraines, myofascial pain syndrome, somatization, and sleep-onset disorder—all of which only describe symptoms and not their cause. No one could put the picture together into a coherent whole.[8] Karen felt she was not being taken seriously and that no one was in control. When doctors would tell her that her symptoms were due to "stress," she felt even more helpless and felt blamed for her own suffering.[9] Meanwhile, doctors groaned when they saw her name on their schedules; some distanced themselves ("Call me in six months"), and others questioned the legitimacy of her complaints.

Then one day an X-ray of Karen's left ankle looked different from the previous ones. Her ankle joint showed signs of inflammation and destruction of the cartilage, just as one would see in rheumatoid arthritis. Now Karen had a disease that could be seen, with pathological changes. Well, sort of. Her blood tests remained normal; she didn't have evidence of any of the known rheumatologic conditions that could explain her joint destruction. She was again left in limbo. She tried increasingly potent (and potentially toxic) medications.[10] While she improved, she also had severe side effects. Once, she developed an infected ulcer on her right ankle that was resistant to antibiotics and continued to fester. Eventually she had prosthetic joints in her knees and right hip and surgery on her wrists, elbow, and shoulder. Still, she walked with a limp and couldn't lift anything heavier than ten pounds. Narcotics, physical therapy, acupuncture, herbal medicines and nutritional supplements, meditation, and psychotherapy were all somewhat helpful, but overall, her trajectory was worsening. She became despondent and hopeless. Her marriage crumbled. I once took a biopsy of her ankle ulcer and on her way home she started to bleed from the biopsy site. She returned to my office, in tears, saying, "I can't take this anymore." I applied pressure, elevated her leg, put in another stitch, and the bleeding stopped. That was the easy part; fixing the wound didn't even begin to touch her suffering.

Patients such as Karen are humbling to clinicians. She had no definite diagnosis. For reasons no one understood, she seemed to get every possible complication from her treatments and didn't heal as well as other patients. No one could untangle the degree to which the causes of her disability and suffering were physical, psychological, or social. The only clear thing was that her suffering was intense. With each downturn, Karen's illness affected me personally. The more ill and depressed she became, the more helpless I felt. I began to dread our visits.

BEYOND HELPLESSNESS

Then, things changed for me in ways that I am still trying to reconstruct. I realized that it wasn't Karen herself who made me feel helpless. Rather, my feeling of helplessness was rooted in an expectation I had of myself—that I could somehow fix something that would then make her suffering abate. When I couldn't fix things, I felt adrift, uncomfortable. The mindful moment was when I simply allowed myself to *feel* helpless and not push that particularly unpleasant feeling away.

Trying to build a wall between myself and her misery would do no good, nor would blaming myself or anyone else. I realized that *feeling* helpless was okay as long as it alerted me to the need to take a fresh look, to adopt a beginner's mind. So I started asking myself questions: Is there something I'm not seeing? Can I take another perspective? Can I be more present with her without being consumed by her despair? At times, the thing to "do" was to do nothing, not reassure, not fix. By temporarily setting aside my need to fix, I could witness her suffering and share her uncertainty, her ambivalence, her hope. The physical exams I performed at each visit became gestures of solidarity as well as a search for pathology.

Doctors are most comfortable fixing things, and I am no exception. We are trained to first identify something gone awry—a symptom such as pain, anxiety, or even existential distress, or a symptomless disease such as hypertension—then to try to restore the patient to a prior state of health using medications, surgery, or behavioral means. Some of Karen's issues were simply unfixable. Surgery would never restore her joints to their pre-arthritis state of twenty years before. Other treatments had backfired, the side effects outweighing any benefit.

It's understandable that doctors pay more attention to health concerns that they feel they can treat effectively. But when the physician's only tool is a diagnose-and-treat approach, he is at risk of being blind to the full range of a patient's suffering. Instead of looking at the patient as a whole person, physicians often view a patient as the sum of the problems that they can recognize, diagnose, and fix.

Months later, Karen began to improve. Her skin infections resolved, her ulcers healed, and she lost much of the weight she had gained; she had a relatively uncomplicated left-hip replacement surgery and could walk without a limp for the first time in years. After a two-month hiatus, she came into the office, beaming and radiant, and the dark look of despair was gone. She was dressed with simple elegance, wearing her own handmade jewelry. I was thunderstruck. I had never, in all the years I had cared for her, seen her so energized and hopeful.

She announced that she had stopped nearly all of her medicines for pain, depression, and insomnia. She decided to leave her (second) husband and felt stronger for having done so. She had taken charge of her life and had found meaning in her existence. "What's changed?" I asked. I was intrigued when she attributed her transition in large part to the support she'd received from me and my colleagues. I was puzzled, so I asked her again, and she said that more important than any particular treatment was that she had felt seen and accompanied—by me and others on her clinical team. She felt that she was never alone. Rather than take this as flattery, I tried to understand why. I pressed her to articulate her experience. In part, her recovery had to do with my recognizing her intentions and goals and supporting her as she tried to refocus her energies and reclaim those parts of her life that were still available to her— even when her symptoms were at their worst. Her words *refocusing* and *reclaiming* stayed with me.[11] "I also like that you are realistic," she said. "You tell me the truth about my illness, but still give me a reason to hope." She appreciated that whenever she voiced opinions about her care, I'd consider them seriously. But perhaps most surprising to me was when she told me how she felt both frightened *and* reassured when I said, "I don't know." "At least," she said, "I knew you were being honest."

A SHORT, SLOW WALK

Tony Back is an oncologist and palliative care physician in Seattle.[12] Together we've been looking at how doctors can better respond to suffering. Recently, Tony has explored what happens when physicians feel helpless. Helplessness is the dark side of the diagnose-and-treat approach—your heart sinks, you feel like a failure.

Tony points out that helplessness is angst provoking, but can also be instructive.[13] The feeling of wanting to turn away and ignore that which one cannot fix can also be a warning sign: "Stop. Wait a minute. This situation demands another approach. Turn toward suffering, not away. Listen deeply so that you can know and accompany the patient and help the patient feel understood."[14] The novelist Henry James calls it placing an "empty cup of attention" between yourself and the patient.[15] The physician-poet Jack Coulehan calls it "compassionate solidarity."[16] In practice, it means saying, "I want to know how you're doing." The point is to check in. The message for physicians is that your negative feelings—despair, confusion, fear, and angst—are an invitation to explore what irks you, to investigate what you'd rather avoid. No one likes feeling helpless. But by turning toward such uncomfortable feelings, rather than shutting them down, I become more effective as a doctor and feel more alive as a human being.

Patients value feeling supported in this way, knowing that I'm willing and able to turn toward them when they are suffering and treat them as whole persons, even under the direst circumstances, whether or not treatments have been effective. This doesn't always require much on my part. For patients who have trouble walking or who are in pain, for instance, I make a point of walking with them the ten yards from the examination room to the reception desk. I accompany them. Granted, it takes a few extra seconds, time that I could spend doing a physical exam, ordering tests. Tacitly, I am sending a message of understanding, nonabandonment, and patience. People want to know that their doctors will accompany them in this way, even if they are only able to walk slowly. For me, that short, slow walk is a contemplative practice, not unlike the Zen practice of slow-walking meditation that punctuates periods of sitting. I become an empathic witness to patients' suffering.

Turning toward suffering means seeing each patient as a person. I come to know what is unique about her, what strengths she has, why she goes on fighting the illness, what underlies her tendency to become dependent on narcotics. Turning toward suffering is "looking into the patient's eyes"[17] rather than just at the diseased body part or a computer screen, entering the landscape of her suffering rather than being a detached observer. Practically speaking, I ask patients about their day, what they can and cannot do, and what their kids need to help them with. These questions don't take long and give me a glimpse of what life is like and what matters most; they often provide clues to the diagnosis and how I can help.

As physicians, we expect patients to tell us when they are suffering and what it's like. But many don't. Instead, patients assume that if something is important, the doctor will ask, or that we don't want to hear, or that we'll think they're complaining or being too demanding. Mindful of patients' reticence, my Rochester colleague and mentor Tim Quill teaches clinicians to ask patients routinely, "What's the worst part of all this?" Rather than presumptuously assuming that he understands, he might say, "I can only begin to imagine . . . ," then he'll ask for more details. Sometimes, at the right moment, he stays silent, letting the patient know that some things cannot be spoken but can nevertheless be shared.[18] Tim is matter-of-fact, open, curious. His willingness to ask indicates that he has something to learn about the patient's suffering from the patient herself, and that he will be able to tolerate what he hears.

Clinicians get little training in how to step out of the comfortable role of diagnostician and accompany patients in this way. Accompanying is particularly important with the patients I don't understand and those who, on the surface, I don't particularly like—those who yell at me, don't tell the truth, or complain then reject the help I offer. Like anyone else, I can feel angry and frustrated, but trying to understand patients in a deeper way—truly seeing them—usually makes caring for them less difficult. When being mindful, I recognize that my irritation is, in part, a signal that I don't understand them—or myself—well enough. My capacity to respond to the suffering of any patient depends on how well I can recognize that my imaginative projection of what the patient is experiencing is just that and no more.

I first learned about this kind of projection during my residency when I was caring for a nineteen-year-old who was on a ventilator in the ICU. He had been diagnosed with meningitis and had complications that included pneumonia and respiratory failure, a scenario with about a 50 percent mortality rate. Gradually, he recovered. He became more alert well before he could be taken off the ventilator and began writing notes. He seemed to tolerate frequent blood draws, suctioning, and invasions of his privacy. He was engaging and had a sweet smile that won the hearts of the medical and nursing staff. He won my heart too. Every day that he was doing well, I felt energized; with each setback, disheartened. I would dream about him at night—anxiety dreams (*Oh, no, I forgot to check his potassium. . . .*) as well as redemption dreams (imagining him playing soccer, free from any signs of disease).

When the tube came out, he could talk again. He still had that same sweet smile, but he was not the person I had imagined. He was immature, demanding, and ungrateful, treating his parents and the staff poorly. He demanded more and more narcotics, perhaps enjoying the brief high they produced. He complained incessantly about the food (here, I did have some sympathy). I was disillusioned. He didn't seem to be following the script—he wasn't the kind, grateful, thoughtful kid I had imagined him to be.

Then I realized to my dismay that I had fabricated an identity for him, an image that hardly any nineteen-year-old could live up to. I was overinvolved. I began to wonder why, then realized that my fabrication obscured a deep fear I had. He was not that far from my own age, and his near-death experience reminded me of the tenuousness of life, the fragility of health. I created a story so that I didn't need to see his vulnerability, or my own.

REFOCUSING AND RECLAIMING

People who are ill seek to make sense of their experience. At the end of life, people who have been disconnected from family often wish to reconnect. Pride, money, and achievements often matter less. People often construct illness stories that give value and honor to the experience of having been ill.[19]

With illnesses that are chronic, debilitating, or difficult to explain, some—but not all—patients seek meaning and coherence. Amid the terror of decline, these patients are uninterested in merely coping; they seek to thrive despite the brutality and unpredictability of their disease. While I believe that few people truly feel grateful for having contracted a serious illness, some feel grateful for the lessons and courage that illness has given them. They feel that they've grown. Witnessing these realizations brings tears to my eyes; I feel a sense of privilege when I see patients refocusing and reclaiming their lives.

Not every patient is interested in refocusing and reclaiming. But I've seen it enough to know that I need to recognize it and nudge it along when I can. Healing becomes a shared project. Patients who wish to approach their illnesses in this way are extraordinary; you cannot force it. Too often, I have heard clinicians and family members exhort patients to "fight" their illnesses, as if they were engaging in a crusade against evil, or to see illness as bringing them closer to God. Sometimes people urge patients to "accept" their illness, as if that final stage in Elisabeth Kübler-Ross's five stages of dying is a value universally shared.[20] It isn't. While some patients may reach an inflection point where they comfortably shift from curative treatments to comfort and palliation, others derive meaning from raging "against the dying of the light."[21] Expectations that patients should somehow transcend their illnesses can burden them with a sense of moral failure that compounds the insults of the disease.

LEARNING TO LISTEN

A family physician colleague, Lucy Candib, has worked for her entire career with indigent and working-class populations in Worcester, Massachusetts, many of whom have experienced abuse, violence, and deprivation. She hears about horrific experiences, examines scarred bodies, and documents what she hears and sees in the hope that it won't happen again to this person, or to anybody else. She is a passionate advocate for those who lack a voice in society, especially for people who seek health care in the aftermath of a life trauma. Candib believes that clinicians should "treat patients' experience as testimony,"[22] verifying and legitimating the personal (if not absolute) truth of each patient's story. Suffering is personal; we all experience it differently. There is no test, no meter, no scale. Treating patients' experience as testimony means respecting a patient's wish to be heard—on her own terms, not anyone else's. This resonates with me, in part because it sets the conditions from which compassion can emerge.

8

The Shaky State
of Compassion

Early in my third year of medical school, I learned of the writings of George Engel. As I mentioned in chapter 1, Engel was the prominent internist and psychoanalyst who formulated a "biopsychosocial model" of care.[1] I wrote to him about my frustrations as a medical student. He shared with me his view that medical institutions, overly preoccupied with technological advances, had forced the human dimensions of medicine to the edges. That was certainly my experience. Engel suggested that I come to Rochester, where the institutional climate was different. In my training in family medicine and subsequent fellowships with him and several of his protégés, I saw a way to achieve what Engel called "being scientific in the human domain."[2]

Engel had an extraordinary capacity to connect with and know other human beings. Patients would meet him for the first time and reveal themselves in ways that provided clues to their medical diagnoses while also creating a human bond. Engel would *look* curious, with a quizzical gaze. He'd ask, "What happened next?" and "What were you thinking when you did that?" and "You mentioned your daughter. What did she suggest? Did it help?" and "What were they doing when your symptoms started?" He'd keep asking until he got a full visual picture of the patient's home, her family, her habits, and her ideas about what was going on. He'd say, "I wonder . . . ," and you'd *feel* a sense of wonder. Patients felt understood.

Engel's approach was radically different from how most of us typically have a social conversation. Maybe you describe an event or a feeling ("When I threw my back out, it was the worst pain of my life"), and your friend responds with a comment, an interpretation, or a question, or she might mention a personal situation that she considers similar to yours ("Yeah, I was in the hospital with a gallbladder attack last year—that was the worst"). This kind of back-and-forth can instill a sense of shared experience: "Wow, she knows what pain is like too." But it can also flop. The other person's story can make you clam up if it doesn't resonate, if you don't feel understood: "What's a slipped disk compared to a gallbladder attack?" you think, irritated.

Engel liked to say that what patients want most is to know and understand what is happening to them and to feel known and understood. Known, not judged. Deep listening is the first step toward compassion. But deep listening is also important for another reason: it is essential to avoiding miscommunications and errors in clinical care. Sometimes when I find myself in a puzzling or challenging situation, I can almost hear Engel's voice in my head, guiding me to listen more deeply, to adopt his inquiring, curious smile.

Deep listening is a form of contemplative practice; it can be taught and learned. In workshops, for example, I'll ask physicians to write and share stories. First, I ask them to select an important event from their professional lives—it could be a moment of connection or it could be a time when things went wrong. Then they take a few minutes to write about it—what happened, who was there, what made it memorable, and whether they were able to make a difference in a positive way. Participants pair off and tell (or read) their story to a partner, who has been instructed to be an attentive listener, and to be aware of—but avoid acting on—an impulse to offer interpretations, advice, or judgments, or to talk about their own experiences. Rather, the listener should contribute only to encourage the storyteller to elaborate, ask clarifying and reflective questions, and explore the storyteller's experience.

While this kind of listening sounds simple, it isn't, especially for physicians, who have been socialized to assume a dominant role in clinical conversations (physicians account for 60 to 80 percent of the talking during an office visit).[3] It takes practice. But, for most people, the feeling of having been listened to—deeply and without judgment—is validating.

SUFFERING WITH

While compassion—"suffering with"—has always been considered a virtue for clinicians (or anyone else), little has been written for physicians about how to cultivate it. Some think of compassion as innate; you either have it or you don't. But we have all seen people who are compassionate under some circumstances but not under others.[4] I've also seen, in students and colleagues, how compassion can grow or wither during one's career.

Compassion is in short supply. Beth Lown, an internist at Harvard's Mount Auburn Hospital and medical director of the Schwartz Center for Compassionate Healthcare, surveyed 800 recently hospitalized patients and 510 physicians in 2011. While 85 percent of patients and 76 percent of physicians said that compassion is "very important" to successful medical treatment, only 53 percent of patients and 58 percent of physicians said that the health care system generally provides compassionate care.[5] And compassion, like presence, is not doled out equitably. Doctors, like most people, tend to be more compassionate toward those whose illnesses they consider legitimate, and less so for those perceived to be at fault for their situation—those who smoke, are obese, or engage in risky sexual behaviors. When physicians lack compassion—or the ability to express it—they inadvertently add to the burden of patients' suffering.

In his landmark experiments about obedience to authority,[6] psychologist Stanley Milgram demonstrated how fragile compassion can be. In one experiment, an authority figure instructed research participants to give electric shocks of increasing strength to a "student" as part of an "experiment on learning." Unbeknownst to the participants, these were mock electric shocks and the "students" were trained actors. Milgram found that the participants were obedient, even though they experienced obvious distress at delivering the shocks. Many gave shocks in the "lethal" range when instructed to do so and continued even when the "student" repeatedly asked that the experiment be stopped. The participants were debriefed after the study and were clearly troubled by their actions.[7] It took so little for them to leave their compassion in the parking lot.

Even those who have the highest aspirations to act compassionately do so only under certain conditions. In the now-famous 1973 Darley and Batson "Jerusalem to Jericho" study, divinity students were instructed to prepare a talk about the biblical parable of the Good Samaritan, a virtuous man who chose to assist a stranger who had been beaten and left for dead on the side of a road.[8] The experimenters placed a shabbily dressed person—obviously in need—slumped by the path that the students took to get to the lecture hall across campus. Half were told they had ample time; the other half were told to hurry or they'd be late. Those in a hurry were much less likely to stop to assist the man in need.

Medical journals frequently publish stories about how physicians—who, like the divinity students in the Good Samaritan study, think of themselves as compassionate—have acted in uncaring ways they later found disturbing. They inflicted pain, did not take the extra moment with a distressed family member, or were rude with a difficult patient. Recently I read a brutally honest story in a medical journal in which an otherwise conscientious physician found himself cutting patients short during an afternoon clinic session so that he could finish on time. Later, he realized that he was doing so because he wanted to arrive refreshed and relaxed for a prestigious lecture he was about to give.[9] The author, a rheumatologist, is a passionate advocate for effective communication in medicine and does research on quality of care. Ironically, I have found myself in exactly the same situation—for example, prior to a dinner with a visiting professor promoting humanism in health care.

CULTIVATING COMPASSION

Up until now, it hasn't been clear what it might take to change this shaky state of compassion. Exhortations to be more compassionate don't work. Compassion isn't a "muscle" that is reliably developed as a result of caring for the sick; some physicians become more cynical and unkind.

Roshi Joan Halifax, anthropologist and Zen Buddhist teacher, has worked with the dying, with prison populations, and with others at the extremes of life. She writes about how compassion is both "contingent and emergent."[10] By contingent, she means that compassion appears in individuals under certain conditions; none of us is intrinsically compassionate all the time. For compassion to emerge, we have to create the right conditions. These conditions have to do with our inner landscape—our own emotional life, attitudes, and self-awareness—and the outer environment, the institutions in which we work. She points out that compassion is cultivated; it isn't a product that can be manufactured. A good gardener cannot make plants grow; she can only coax them to grow and flourish by cultivating the soil and providing nutrients and water. Similarly, compassion doesn't spring from the earth unbidden and it doesn't easily submit to checklists and industrial models of health care. Compassion is also emergent in that it may manifest in surprising and unpredictable ways—through words, small gestures, advocacy, even silence. The challenge is to create those conditions in which compassion is *most likely* to arise, but not necessarily to expect it to manifest the same way each time.

INGREDIENTS OF COMPASSION

Compassion is the triad of *noticing another's suffering, resonating with their suffering in some way*, and then *acting* on behalf of another person. Research suggests that awareness of our inner states can help us recognize the inner states of others.[11] Some of the same neural circuits are activated when we witness pain as when we experience our own.[12] When we are distressed, we feel it first in the body; we do the same when taking in the distress of others, mapping their experiences onto our own, and feeling pain in response to theirs.[13]

Yet the feelings and sensations that patients elicit in me are not the same ones that patients experience; I resonate with their pain, but it's not the same. This resonance is the second ingredient of compassion—the "suffering with" part. A boundary gets blurred and you hurt too. But if I assume that what I am feeling is exactly what the patient is feeling, I would be wrong much of the time. I've made the mistake of mentioning to patients who've had kidney stones that I've had them too. Some patients take this as an empathic gesture, which leads to a sense of shared experience, but more often my self-disclosure falls flat; patients want me to understand *their* unique experience. They're interested in *their* kidney stones and aren't particularly interested in mine. Although I might think I understand their pain, their bland responses to my revelation confirm that I'm off the mark. My time is better spent asking about what it was like for them.[14]

The third ingredient of compassion is *action* to reduce another's suffering. Like most people, particularly those in helping professions, physicians often experience meaning and purpose when they do things to benefit others; compassion nourishes the healer. Engaging in compassionate action, we release endogenous opioids, which attenuate our own pain; dopamine, which promotes a sense of reward; and oxytocin, which generates feelings of caring, affiliation, and belonging.[15] I suspect this reward response may be part of the reason clinicians work long hours throughout their careers and continue to work into their seventies and eighties, long after people in other professions have retired.

But if compassion is its own reward—if it fills clinicians with a deep sense of purpose and well-being—then why is it in such short supply in health care? The answer has to do with the second of the three ingredients: resonating. When I resonate emotionally with another person's suffering, I experience distress, a discomfort within. If I feel that I can do something to relieve the patient's distress quickly, my own distress also dissipates. But if it's not possible—if I lack the skills or if it's going to take a long time—there's a natural human tendency to withdraw, to pull away in self-protection. Mindfulness, here, is observing, understanding, and regulating my own emotional reactions so I can reliably sustain presence in the face of a patient's distress—and my own.

THE PARADOX OF EMPATHY

Every medical school in North America now has a communication skills course. Typically students are tested on their empathy through exercises with actors trained to portray patients in distress. But these efforts don't seem to have had enough of an effect on the seemingly inevitable decline in empathy during medical training.[16]

Empathy, like compassion, has many definitions, but at its basis is a bodily, emotional, and cognitive insight into another person's emotional life.[17] This insight can be experienced and communicated in a cool and detached way ("If I understand correctly, this has been very difficult for you"), a welling up of emotion ("This is just awful"), or a bodily sensation, such as feeling your heart sinking or a lump in your throat. In medical education, students are taught to recognize and name another's distress as an emotion without experiencing that state themselves—"I can see that you're feeling afraid" or "You're telling me that you were furious with him" or even "Very unsettling, all this uncertainty." This kind of empathy is accurate, but can be chilly.

This cool cognitive empathy is not always what patients want. They want a sense of emotional connection and caring; they want the physician to be warm and attuned to what they are feeling. However, it is a delicate balance for physicians. Sharing their personal feelings with patients is not always helpful and sometimes diverts the conversation away from what concerns the patient.[18] Mindful clinicians are present, attuned, and empathic without appropriating the focus of attention from their patients to themselves.

Juggling three "balls"—being empathically attuned to another person's emotions, being attuned to your own emotions, and acting on the other person's behalf—has been the focus of research by psychologists Carl Batson and Nancy Eisenberg for the past forty years.[19] Using a variety of laboratory experiments, they have found that when we understand and assimilate another person's emotions, we all reach a proverbial fork in the road. One path leads to self-protection: You say and do things to lower your own anxiety. You rationalize your actions. What you do may or may not help the other person. In short, you are focused on yourself and your own feelings. The other path leads to "pro-social" behavior, acts that relieve the patient's distress through words, medications, surgery, or just by being present. It can be an expression of heartfelt connection with the patient—what physician Michael Kearney calls "exquisite empathy"[20]—or compassionate action that directly relieves the patient's suffering.

In a series of experiments, Olga Klimecki at the University of Geneva and her colleagues set out to explore whether she could train people to be more compassionate.[21] She based her training on Batson and Eisenberg's model. First, she trained a group of participants to recognize and resonate with the emotions of others. While in a functional MRI scanner, the participants then watched videos that depicted human suffering and later completed surveys that measured empathy and personal distress. Then, in a second session, she led them in "kindness" meditation practices to evoke feelings of benevolence, kindness, and caring toward themselves and others (friends, "neutral" persons, and "difficult" persons), a practice designed to evoke compassion.[22] Again, the participants were scanned and completed surveys. The results confirmed Batson and Eisenberg's predictions: those trained only to resonate with others—and without skills to translate that resonance into compassion—felt more emotionally distressed; their brain scans showed greater activation in areas of the brain known to be associated with distress and vicarious pain.[23] After receiving just one day of compassion training, these same people had a different neural "signature." They felt energized and had a more positive sense of self. The scans of those who received compassion training showed that their "reward pathways"[24] were activated and the "distress pathways" were no longer active.

These are experiments in a laboratory and present crude models of how the brain—and the mind—works in the real world. But they are revealing in terms of how we train doctors.[25] I finally understood why training physicians to be more sensitive and to resonate with patients' emotional distress—a good thing—can lead to emotional exhaustion and burnout. In fact, when I've surveyed students and residents, some of those who score highest on empathy are sometimes the most burned out. They experience secondary—or vicarious—trauma from having assimilated the suffering of others. For years, I had been training medical students, residents, and practicing physicians to name and acknowledge the patient's feelings, by saying things like "Now I have a better understanding of how much pain you're in." Was this approach all wrong? Could it be that too much empathy was toxic? We had been training our students to share emotions and take the patient's perspective, but had failed to help them be aware of and manage their own strong feelings. Feeling traumatized, they disconnected, assumed a stance of cool objectivity, avoided getting involved. Which is to say that training in empathy is a good thing, but it goes only so far. It's now clear that we also need to train physicians to be compassionate, not only for the sake of their patients, but because compassionate action seems to relieve the emotional tension that is inevitable when we try to imagine the experience of another. It's an antidote to burnout.

We know now that it is possible to train clinicians to be more compassionate, an idea that would have been considered radical just a few years ago. Yet, the emotional "climate" of the health care institutions within which doctors work is typically unsupportive, hardly providing a model of compassion that clinicians can emulate with their patients. To provide compassionate care, we have to address institutional climate and values. Consider the alternative. Empathy—and compassion—are doomed to decline if we continue to neglect the emotional lives of physicians, if we fail to provide the conditions under which they can learn to regulate their emotions, develop mental stability, and have the right kind of equanimity—an engaged equanimity in which clinicians are present with—but not consumed by—patients' emotional needs. And it's not just physicians; "compassion fatigue" is as much of a problem among nurses and other health professionals.

TRAINING IN COMPASSION

But how?

When I learned about metta meditation—sometimes called loving-kindness meditation or compassion practice—it initially struck me as insufferably New Age. I couldn't imagine how dreamy voices, pictures of lotuses, and invitations to a "revolutionary art of happiness"[26] could possibly appeal to hard-edged physicians.

Metta is a Pali word that translates as "friendship" and "kindness," a sincere wish for the welfare and genuine happiness of others. Metta is an attitude that the practitioner aspires to bring to all beings, without exception—so-called nonreferential or unconditional compassion—akin to Aristotle's concept of *philia*, or "brotherly love."[27] If you take the view that humans have the capacity for compassion but are hindered by a distorted view of the world, then it is possible to remove those hindrances through practice.

The first time I experienced it, I was at a workshop. During the guided meditation, the teacher instructed us to imagine ourselves and our positive attributes, then to extend kindness to ourselves, then a "benefactor," a friend, a "neutral person," a "difficult person," and finally "all beings." We were asked to enact silently, in our minds, a series of phrases, first directed toward ourselves: "May I be free from danger, may I be happy, may I be healthy, may I live with ease." Then, to others, in turn: "May they be free from danger, may they be happy, may they be healthy, may they live with ease." And so on.

I took some solace when I learned that compassion practice has been part of meditation traditions for over twenty-five hundred years. But could you really train people to be kind, to befriend, to *care*? Or was this exercise an indulgence, helping well-educated, privileged healthy people feel good about themselves? Somewhat skeptical, I went along with the exercise, trying to keep an open mind. I noticed that it was more difficult to wish myself well than to direct kindness toward a friend. This certainly was revealing in how difficult it is for clinicians to care for themselves. I wondered what a "benefactor" meant to me, and how I had expressed my gratitude for my benefactors' selfless actions. It helped me appreciate how many people had helped me to get where I am. When I was asked to imagine standing beside a "difficult person" and wishing him well, I became more curious about my interactions with people whom I regarded as difficult and began to recognize that their presence was teaching me something helpful too. I found myself feeling deeply grateful—to others and to myself. Being in a room with others, all of whom were working on cultivating something positive, was powerful—it created a sense of community and shared purpose. What had seemed to be a rather odd and forced exercise began to make sense.[28]

Since then, at least one research study has distinguished the neural fingerprint of compassion practice from other forms of contemplative practice. Studying a group of novice meditators for nine months, psychologist Tania Singer's research group at the Max Planck Institute found that compassion practice led to activation of the inferior parietal cortex, the dorsolateral prefrontal cortex, and the nucleus accumbens—demonstrating links between the "reward circuit" in the brain and the parts of the brain that have to do with understanding and resonating with the feelings of others, and the ability to regulate our own emotions (what is commonly called emotional intelligence).[29] While you don't need a functional MRI scan to "prove" that bestowing kindness on yourself and other human beings is a good thing, this line of research[30] is tantalizing now that evidence suggests that through practice people can act more altruistically and expand their emotional compass.

9

When Bad Things Happen

Angela Bradowski had over three hundred pounds on her five-foot-three-inch frame. For the first two years after I diagnosed her with diabetes, she controlled her disease with oral medications. Then her blood sugars started climbing from the 100s to the 200s, then the 300s. I didn't see her for a few months, and when she came back, her blood sugar was nearly 500. When it gets above 600 or so, people are at risk for coma and even death.

Angela had all of the classic signs of poorly controlled diabetes—insatiable thirst, frequent and copious urination, weakness, and blurry vision. I started her on a long-acting insulin (glargine), otherwise known as Lantus. Normally insulin doses range between thirty and eighty units per day, and patients with insulin resistance may need doses in excess of one hundred units. But Angela didn't seem to respond, and with each visit I increased her insulin even further.

I started to feel out of my element when her Lantus dose exceeded one hundred units twice daily. I consulted the medical literature and called a diabetologist. He had had a couple of patients who had needed doses of over four hundred units a day, and some cases in the literature documented patients receiving close to a thousand units. Emboldened, I kept increasing the dose, and eventually Angela was giving herself four hundred units twice a day, and still her sugar was out of control.

I asked Angela about her diet, medications, and physical activity—the usual questions—yet I was baffled. Nothing seemed to explain the situation. She didn't eat all that much. She didn't exercise, but that wouldn't explain her extraordinary resistance to insulin. The most common explanation—not taking her insulin—didn't seem to apply. She had the skin marks to prove it, and she had been refilling her vials of insulin on schedule.

Occasionally people are more sensitive to one formulation of insulin than another. With that in mind and on the advice of the diabetologist, I switched her insulin from long-acting to intermediate-acting (NPH) insulin. Not knowing what would happen, I started her on eighty units twice a day, one-fifth of her previous dose. I was hoping that the more rapid onset might control her blood sugar more effectively. It seemed to be worth a try.

The next day she was hospitalized with a stroke. She was found unconscious at home and her blood sugar was zero when the ambulance arrived. By the time I got to the hospital, she was beginning to wake up; she was drowsy, but couldn't move her left side. In the emergency room, George, her husband, was waiting for news about Angela's condition. He told me that he had been worrying about her because, unbeknownst to me, she had been slaking her unquenchable thirst with three two-liter bottles of sweetened iced tea every day. My heart sank. Now it all made sense. I did a quick calculation—at least two thousand calories in addition to whatever else she was eating.

When diabetes is out of control, glucose doesn't get into the cells and stays in the blood, making people urinate copiously and frequently to try to get rid of the sugar. As a result, they get dehydrated and thirsty. Insulin also makes you hungry and gain weight. Angela's craving for liquids and sweets was insatiable—the more she took in, the worse it got. I had asked what she ate every day, and I had asked about soft drinks, but I hadn't thought to ask about iced tea—and she didn't volunteer it. Because Lantus acts slowly, she could take in enough sugar to keep up with the insulin, and then some. In essence, I was prescribing what for most of us would be a lethal dose of insulin, and she was rescuing herself from hypoglycemia with her own form of resuscitation, which then would send her blood sugar skyrocketing. But, with the switch to NPH insulin, this could no longer work. NPH has a more rapid onset and she couldn't keep up, no matter how fast she might drink—even though the dose was lower. She almost died—at least in part from following my instructions.

I vacillated between being furious with her for not telling me an important piece of information and being furious at myself for not having done a more thorough nutritional assessment. She certainly had the opportunity to tell me, but perhaps she felt she needed to hide it, or perhaps it never occurred to her. While I didn't bear sole responsibility for the situation, neither did she. It was somewhere in the middle. She had seen other physicians and the nurse-practitioner on our primary care team. None of them asked either. In that sense, our health care team failed her. One could even say that the larger health care system failed her. She had many life stressors and a long list of physical and psychological conditions, and the fifteen-minute visits that were allotted to her didn't allow enough time to address them all—or even come close. Her insurance covered only a one-time visit to a dietitian, and she had used that up. Perhaps with more time for each visit, or a more sustained relationship with a nutritionist, her iced tea consumption might have been disclosed.

Angela was fortunate. Over the next two days she improved, with seemingly little residual damage. It's remarkable that she survived at all. She went home a few days later on low doses of NPH insulin—and no iced tea. She was scared and never wanted to have something like that happen again. She controlled her diabetes effectively from that point on. She lost weight. I told her that I felt bad about having prescribed a dose of insulin that resulted in a major scare. It's remarkable how forgiving some patients can be. She was grateful to be alive.

After the dust settled, I mentioned the event to a trusted colleague. In an attempt to be supportive, he was all too eager to absolve me of any responsibility before having assimilated the details of the situation, saying that I had done nothing wrong and that the responsibility was the patient's. Strikingly, for him it didn't even register as an error, yet I felt traumatized. In fact, if you ask most physicians whether they have made a significant error during their medical careers, they will more likely than not say no, they haven't. Yet over one hundred thousand patients die each year as a result of medical errors, mostly preventable, and hundreds of thousands more experience nonfatal errors and near misses.[1] Experts on medical errors would define Angela's as a "potentially preventable" error—a near miss.

FATAL MISTAKES

Other errors don't have such positive outcomes. Most dramatic are medication errors and surgical errors. Several years ago I discharged Kathryn Wolk from the hospital with a prescription for methotrexate—a powerful immunosuppressive medication to help control her symptoms of lupus. She was transferred from the hospital to a nursing home under the care of the nursing home physician. Somewhere in the transition to the nursing home, someone—it's not clear who—wrote that Kathryn should be receiving three pills daily. The correct dose—the dose she was receiving in the hospital—was three pills once a week. The incorrect prescription wasn't noticed for months until I received a report from the nursing home. I was furious and incredulous. How could this happen? By that time she had developed pulmonary fibrosis, irreversible scarring of the lungs caused by methotrexate toxicity. She died several weeks later.

Kathryn's daughter was also a patient of mine. I had to explain. "Everyone feels very badly that this happened, myself included. Kathryn clearly got the wrong dose. It was a terrible miscommunication." This explanation didn't sit well with Kathryn's daughter. "Why didn't anyone notice?" she inquired. I was honest: "I scoured the records—at least the ones I have access to—and I can't figure it out. The discharge medication list said three pills weekly rather than three pills daily." She asked, "You mean to tell me that she might have lived longer—maybe a couple of years? Do you think that I should talk to a lawyer?" If there's anything to make a doctor feel on the defensive, to feel judged and inadequate, it is the threat of litigation.

Here, a grief-stricken family member is trying to make sense of a complex series of events. She was puzzled, not only by how the events could have occurred, but also by my response. I felt devastated, but I had been counseled not to say anything that might implicate myself or anyone else. Kathryn's daughter, like most people in these kinds of situations, wanted to know the answers to several simple questions: Did I or didn't I personally make a mistake? Am I really sorry? Shouldn't I apologize? Will this kind of mistake happen again?[2] Even though I knew that I had written the correct order on Kathryn's discharge paperwork, I was questioning myself—did I *really* communicate clearly? Was I really at fault? I was so preoccupied with my own conflicted sense of responsibility that I couldn't be fully present with Kathryn's daughter. I just wanted to hide.

In 2000 the Institute of Medicine published a game-changing report on medical error in which they suggested that most errors in hospitals were problems of institutions, not of individuals.[3] The revelation for most clinicians was that institutions were set up in such a way that errors were inevitable. This radical shift in consciousness impelled health care institutions to enact procedures to reduce errors—especially medication errors and surgical mishaps—through checklists, handoff protocols when patients were transferred to a new unit, team training, and time-outs prior to surgical procedures to assure that important details weren't missed.

The methotrexate disaster occurred a number of years ago, and perhaps tragedies like this are less likely now. But they still happen, and in some cases the solutions designed to prevent future errors, such as electronic health records, create the conditions for a whole new set of errors—for example, those that result from patients being transferred among institutions that have incompatible electronic record systems. Here, the error was a systems failure. It was a demonstration of the "Swiss cheese" model of medical error in which bad things happen when all the holes in the system happen to line up.[4] My intention, though, is not to assign blame or guilt or to propose how these situations could have been avoided or changed. I've already explored how errors happen through inattention, not seeing, not being curious, not having an open mind, not being present—and how the solutions, often unique to each situation, depend on local factors. Here, I am exploring how physicians might approach bad outcomes more mindfully, regardless of their own responsibility.

Physicians generally endorse the approach I took when meeting with Kathryn's family—a measured disclosure and an expression of regret, without falling to pieces emotionally or assuming guilt. Yet when patients sense a lack of heartfelt regret, it only fans the flames of their anger and feelings of abandonment.

Physicians don't apologize because they feel afraid. Lawsuits are just the tip of the iceberg. "Morbidity and mortality" rounds in surgical specialties can be a sadistic ritual in which the guilty party is thrown to the lions; there's no sympathy or support. Even when lawsuits aren't an issue, doctors are afraid to confront their fallibility. When we're afraid, we clam up, which only makes matters worse because patients interpret lack of communication as lack of caring. Most malpractice suits start with a real or perceived error but are carried forward only if patients feel abandoned, if they feel that the doctor hasn't listened or hasn't expressed regret.[5] Research by psychologists, physicians, and attorneys consistently shows that patients want an apology—it improves communication and diffuses anger.[6] One research study even created mock trials; settlements were lower when physicians apologized.[7] By trying to protect themselves, physicians may paradoxically increase their risk of being sued.

With that in mind, most states have enacted "apology laws." These laws, which offer some degree of protection to physicians if they are more fully disclosing about medical errors, have been associated with fewer and smaller malpractice settlements.[8] Yet, physicians still hide, and apologies still don't happen as often and in the way that they should.

THE SECOND VICTIM

With all of the current attention to errors, no one seemed to be paying attention to the inner lives of physicians when things go wrong—the emotional and interpersonal fallout of a bad outcome. In 2007, Amy Waterman, a researcher at Washington University in St. Louis, surveyed 3,171 physicians in the United States and Canada about the aftermath of medical errors and near misses. Of those who reported that they had made errors, most felt traumatized; 61 percent reported that they were more anxious about future errors, and over 40 percent reported loss of confidence, sleeping difficulties, and lower job satisfaction. Even near misses increased stress. I was not surprised that only 10 percent of the physicians surveyed said that their health care organizations were supportive after they or a colleague had made an error; I doubt it's much better now.[9] The emotional climate remains hostile; in general, physicians don't want to hear about one another's errors, and only now are health care institutions recognizing clinicians' psychological trauma.

In a prescient essay in 2000, internist Albert Wu described how physicians can be "second victims" when medical errors happen:

> Virtually every practitioner knows the sickening feeling of making a bad mistake. You feel singled out and exposed—seized by the instinct to see if anyone has noticed. You agonize about what to do, whether to tell anyone, what to say. Later, the event replays itself over and over in your mind. You question your competence but fear being discovered. You know you should confess, but dread the prospect of potential punishment and of the patient's anger.[10]

Wu described the hospital team's reaction to a resident who had misread an electrocardiogram a few hours previously. The patient had pericardial tamponade, a life-threatening situation in which the pericardium—the sac that contains the heart—fills with fluid. The patient was rushed to the operating room in the middle of the night in extremis, a situation that could have been avoided had the

EKG been interpreted correctly. On rounds, the resident's colleagues were stunned and silent, perhaps because they were secretly afraid that they might have made the same mistake in similar circumstances; they were unable to respond with compassion to their classmate's shame.

When I was doing one of my medical school rotations, I was paired with a student who was struggling. He had grown up in a culture where the interpersonal norms were radically different from the environment on the wards of a Boston teaching hospital. When being grilled on rounds, he spoke slowly and modestly—a virtue in his culture—which only invoked the impatience of his superiors. I tried to be supportive, but didn't know how. I had a sense that his experience invoked feelings of shame, but I wasn't sure even about that. He withdrew further. No wonder doctors become emotionally unavailable to their patients—they are beaten into not even being available for themselves.

Even aviation does better. Aviation is not known for being a warm and fuzzy industry; yet after near misses crew members are debriefed, counseled, and given time off. They aren't returned to the workplace until everyone is assured that they've recovered sufficiently.[11] Yet, after being present at a stillbirth, we doctors are expected to go straightaway into the next room to deliver a healthy full-term child. An anesthesiologist, after the death of a patient on the operating table, typically will move on to the next case with barely five minutes to regroup. Medicine has learned a lot from aviation in terms of checklists, teamwork, and error prevention,[12] but much less about managing the emotional impact of disasters and near misses. Given the imprecision of clinical practice, it's remarkable that doctors should think of themselves as more infallible than pilots. While feedback and debriefing are now more common, support is often brief and superficial. Without tools to deepen self-awareness and without exploring thinking processes and emotions in greater depth, the wounds fester and no one learns. Unexamined exposure to repeated trauma cannot but cause trauma itself.

The consequences of secondary traumatization—being the second victim—weren't talked about much until recently. It has become clear that when things don't go well and doctors don't get the support that they (or anyone) need, they often go down with the ship. They are at greater risk for depression and burnout. They feel badly about themselves and, as a consequence, are distracted and less emotionally available to their patients; they become less empathic. They lose their self-confidence and are more likely to make errors in the future.[13] They fear future humiliations. Too often, despite experiencing strong emotions, they bury their feelings and instead just focus on survival strategies; awareness and mindful responsiveness take a backseat.

REMEMBERING

Physicians remember their mistakes and are haunted by them. They hold them in silence for years, sometimes decades. Their stories reveal their psychological vulnerabilities—unrelenting perfectionism, unforgiving intolerance of error, unease in the face of ambiguity, a desperate need for certainty. While many physicians will acknowledge these vulnerabilities if asked, during everyday practice they usually lurk just outside awareness.

During one workshop, Mark, a psychiatrist, told of a patient who committed suicide with the medications that Mark had prescribed for him the day before. Mark had never told anyone for fear of being chastised for having given the patient a month's supply of pills. Mark had been living with a discomfiting sense of ambiguity about his own role in the tragedy, still having intrusive dreams, waking up in a sweat. Should he have done a more thorough assessment of the patient's suicidality? Should he have prescribed only a week's worth of medication at a time? He lost his self-confidence. One afternoon at the workshop was devoted to errors in medicine—how we respond when things go wrong. Mark put on paper his recollection of what had happened, what he felt in his body at the time, and the accompanying thoughts, feelings, and emotions. Then he spent twenty minutes sharing his narrative with a partner who had been instructed to listen deeply—to suspend judgment and to try to understand and be curious about the situation and Mark's reactions. As difficult as it was to listen with openness without trying to console or offer advice, Mark's partner was able to be present and not avoid or turn away from the painful moments; this invited Mark to do the same. A burden of fear and apprehension was lifted; he was reenergized, more attentive, less afraid of the difficult moments in his practice. He was able to move on. It seemed simple enough, but in the four years since his patient's suicide, there had been no natural place for Mark to disclose and examine his reactions.

I could relate to Mark's story. I also had a patient who committed suicide with medications that I had prescribed that day. My colleagues tried to assuage my guilt without really listening to the impact that event had on me. Everyone just assumed that was part of being a doctor. Get over it. Move on. I later learned that I'm not alone. It is the norm in medicine for colleagues to offer brief words of consolation, then shut down feelings. Yet the wounds fester and never heal; clinicians remain troubled and act in ways that make patients feel that they're not all there. Some physicians—family doctors, surgeons, psychiatrists—have committed suicide in the aftermath of an error. But when doctors are given the chance to address the impact of a bad outcome, they feel a sense of relief. It's no longer a secret. Addressing errors means accepting their imperfections, paving the way for kindness and compassion toward themselves, which can then enable physicians to do their jobs better, less encumbered.

CONFESSIONS

One of my colleagues in Rochester, Suzie Karan, a senior anesthesiologist, is well aware of how rarely errors and near misses are disclosed and discussed. Anesthesiologists administer powerful medications as a matter of course; without ventilators, IVs, and monitors, these medication doses would be lethal. The work of anesthesiologists in the OR is 90 percent routine and 10 percent terror. When things go sour, there is no tolerance for error or delay. Yet errors do happen and until recently there were few opportunities to debrief.

A few years ago, Karan started the "confessions" project, now implemented in residency programs at several medical centers. The project has been remarkably effective in bringing errors to the collective consciousness of the house staff and faculty—not only with an eye to identify the causes and prevent future errors, but also to address the psychological and educational needs of the clinicians involved. The mandatory sessions occur weekly for beginning residents, then several times a year for the more senior residents and staff. Each resident brings an account of an event, printed on an eight-and-a-half-by-eleven page in 12-point Times New Roman font to ensure that the reports are anonymous. They record their recollections and impressions, what happened, who was there, what they did, and how they felt, then fold the page and place it into the "confessions" pile.

Even though the tone of the word *confessions* implies something gone terribly wrong, the residents do sometimes confess something positive, a disaster averted. At the meetings, the confessions, one from each person, are distributed randomly, and the residents, one by one, read them aloud, not knowing who the writer might be. The residents discuss the event and what they can do going forward. Sometimes the discussions are emotional. Whether the disclosure is about a major catastrophe or a near miss or an everyday mishap, the goal is to help the residents grow their ability to self-regulate while building support and camaraderie.

One story was written by a doctor who accidentally spilled an anesthetic medication on the floor. Foolishly, he tried to clean it up himself, and even though he kept as close to the floor as possible to avoid breathing the highly volatile gases, within a minute he became woozy, nearly unconscious. No one discovered him. He got his bearings after several minutes, left the room, and never told anyone. Another resident accidentally gave ten times the dose of an intravenous anesthetic, and while the patient (fortunately) did fine, he never told anyone for fear of being reprimanded. The discussion inspired a collective sense of mindful vigilance and important safety initiatives, all born out of greater self-awareness. I believe that the real power of Karan's project is in changing the culture of medicine from a culture of secrecy to a culture of inquiry, of curiosity, in which clinicians are vigilant not only of their patients but also of themselves. Karan's approach emphasizes collaborative problem solving, forgiveness, and learning—all in one gesture—to help the residents to direct their attention to what matters right now, learning from the past rather than replaying the events over and over; the residents could see the events more clearly without the distractions of self-blame or self-justification.[14]

GRIEF AND LOSS

I admitted Ruth Miller to the palliative care unit. She had been diagnosed just a few weeks before with an unusually aggressive lung cancer, which had already spread to her ribs, spine, and brain. She had started radiation treatments, but things only got worse; she was confused, disoriented, and in considerable pain. I informed Ruth's family—already in shock from the diagnosis—that she likely had only a few weeks, perhaps as long as three months, to live. Her cancer was not of a type that would respond to one of the new targeted chemotherapies, nor to anything else. Family members from different parts of the country were making plans to fly in to visit.

With medications we controlled Ruth's pain and cleared her confusion enough so that she could talk and interact with her family over the next few days. She was in her best spirits in weeks. Her family left for the evening. Two hours later, David, her nurse, made a routine check, and Ruth wasn't breathing. One of the brain metastases had likely hemorrhaged, sending Ruth into an instant coma followed by respiratory arrest. Nothing could have been done to prevent it even if she had had the most aggressive care possible; hers was a quick and painless demise. David was stunned; he and Ruth's family all thought they had at least a few more days to prepare.

David was grieving but fearless. He had grown close to the family and wanted to be the one to call them. I overheard the conversation. He gave the news. Briefly. Then he waited and listened. He expressed his own sense of sorrow and surprise in a way that I later learned had made the family feel understood. He asked how their last visit with Ruth had been. He explained what would happen next. David's grief was palpable to me; his response, though, was present, attentive, and generous at a time when he himself was in shock. He and I spoke for a few minutes afterward to debrief. His grief triggered compassion rather than self-absorption; he was strong enough to acknowledge and be with his own emotions, yet could set them aside to be present with Ruth's family.

FALLING SHORT AND FALLING APART

Doctors tend to take death, errors, and other bad outcomes as personal setbacks. Perhaps a few Zen masters can consistently approach these kinds of ego-crushing experiences as fodder for growth, but the rest of us need help achieving the fearlessness that is required to look our failures in the eye. It means recognizing the fault lines, allowing ourselves to fall apart just a little bit to feel the pain of failure, but not so much that we become ineffective or overwhelmed. Attention training and other contemplative practices are powerful in part because they help you practice letting go of the need to cement things together.

Grief can be even more intense when clinicians have known patients for months or years. Mitch Porter had seen me for his diabetes for over twenty years. A successful businessman, at age fifty-four he was at the peak of his career. In the past year, he had sold a small business, received a community service award from the local chamber of commerce, and bought a vacation house in Costa Rica. He came to see me because he was having worsening right-flank pain and blood in his urine. I ordered an ultrasound of his kidneys and bladder, expecting to see evidence of a kidney stone. Instead, the ultrasonographer saw a small mass in his kidney and enlarged lymph nodes nearby. Mitch and his partner were terrified and I was filled with dread. I ordered more scans and blood tests to see just how far the cancer had metastasized. The bone scans showed cancer in his spine and nearly every large bone in his body, from his feet to his skull. His lungs were filled with hundreds of metastases, and there was spread to his brain. I started grieving even before he and his family could begin to feel the devastation. I was about to lose someone who had entrusted his well-being to me, and now we were talking weeks.

As the lab and scan results crossed my desk, one by one painting an increasingly lethal picture, I found myself wondering if I could have done something sooner. While trying to be in the present moment, again and again my mind would go in the same circles of self-doubt and self-reassurance. I felt stupid engaging in the seemingly useless exercise of trying to undo the past. I then asked myself, "Is this cycle useful in some way? Where is it directing my attention?" I watched the thoughts rather than labeling them as useless or obsessive, not grasping on to them, not pushing them away. Then the thoughts of self-blame gave way to a deep sadness. Letting go of self-blame didn't mean giving up. Quite the opposite. It energized me to do what needed to be done now, rather than trying to undo the past. I contacted his oncologist and his radiation oncologist to discuss a treatment plan. Having entered into uncertainty and instability with my eyes open, I could clarify what I could and couldn't control.

A SMOKELIKE QUALITY

Leeat Granek is a psychologist in Toronto whose mother died after a twenty-year bout with breast cancer. Granek felt a deep sense of connection with her mother's care team and came to wonder how health professionals deal with their grief when their patients die. So she asked. She interviewed twenty oncologists at different stages in their careers. Although half of their patients will die of their cancer, oncology is a culture in which cure is seen as the goal despite sometimes great odds. Oncologists see their patients frequently. A bond forms. Even when patients have cancers that cannot be cured, many have a reasonable quality of life—for a while.

Then things go sour. Patients lose weight. The chemotherapy stops working. The side effects become more burdensome, outweighing any benefit. Patients get weaker. Oncologists described how they'd drag themselves into patients' rooms, consumed by a sense of failure. They would cry in the car on the way home. Some would excoriate themselves, wondering whether they could have done something differently. Some shut down emotionally. One oncologist said, "It is a very bad thing to become emotionally attached to your patients because *you're* going to suffer." Unexamined grief led some oncologists to offer more aggressive chemotherapy to subsequent patients than they might otherwise have, treatments that lead to more suffering with a negligible chance of improving either quality or quantity of life. Granek was moved by the interviews. She said that the doctors' grief had a "smoke-like quality . . . intangible and invisible . . . pervasive, sticking to the physicians' clothes when they went home after work and slipping under the doors between patient rooms,"[15] a feeling that they couldn't set aside or wash away.

Not all oncologists responded in dysfunctional ways, though. Some were more like David, Ruth's nurse. They described how patients' deaths molded and humbled them, helping them to be more present. Confronting loss made them more careful, more respectful, and less willing merely to accept the status quo. They became activists on their patients' behalf, whether this meant getting approval for a medication that an insurance company didn't want to pay for or spending time talking with a family about how to care for their loved one during his final days. The doctors derived a sense of fulfillment from caring for the dying.

Rachel Rodenbach wanted to find out how and why some oncologists had this capacity for equanimity, advocacy, and activism in the face of death, whereas others didn't.[16] Rachel was a medical student at the time, and now is a resident planning to go into oncology. She sought me as her supervisor for a year-long project, proposing to interview oncology clinicians—doctors, nurse-practitioners, and physician assistants—about their views on their own deaths and how their attitudes influenced their care of patients who were at the end of life. At first I had my doubts. Given how personal these interviews would be, I didn't know how many clinicians would sign up. But Rachel's project struck a chord with them, and the majority of those whom she asked ultimately *did* participate. Despite their impossibly busy schedules, they took the time to talk and reflect. Frequently, the interviews ran over the allotted time; they had a lot to say and found talking to be cathartic.

Rachel first asked the oncologists whether they could accept the idea of their own deaths. Some said that they were completely at peace with their own deaths, and others indicated that they were terrified, but the majority said yes—sort of: "But I've not really had to face it, so I really don't know how I'd feel." They were being self-aware and honest with themselves.

Some reflected on how their sense of peace (or lack thereof) affected their interactions with patients—for example, whether they tended to talk about death directly with patients or whether they tended to use euphemisms or beat around the bush. Some would only discuss death and dying with the patient's family members, sensing their own and the patient's discomfort. Many said that when they were able to be more self-aware, they could bring more of themselves to the patients they were caring for.

Leeat Granek's oncologists, similar to those interviewed by Rachel Rodenbach, saw a need for change in the culture of cancer care; currently, it glorifies the cure and conquest of cancer, treats death as failure, and regards expressions of emotion as a sign of weakness. Yet, oncologists said that they valued training, information, support, and validation to help them deal more effectively with their own grief; they could see that trying to push away painful feelings wasn't an effective way of dealing with them.[17] At Rochester, my colleagues Tim Quill and Michelle Shayne have developed a program to promote reflection and mindfulness for oncologists in training and clinical staff.[18] Six times a year the trainees and clinical staff meet with a senior oncologist, a palliative care specialist, and a clergyman to enhance their awareness of and address the impact of grief and loss on their personal and professional lives. They share stories about patients for whom they cared. They laugh, they cry. Part of the time is set aside for self-care, including meditation. At the end of each session, they hold a moment of silence in remembrance of patients who have died. If so moved, they speak the name of one patient to remember and honor him. It sets a tone that would have been considered radical until recently; it hones clinicians' ability to care for themselves in the service of being more present for patients. It brings awareness of shared humanity and intimacy as well as the relationship between clinicians' vulnerabilities and those of their patients. They realize that feeling and sharing emotions is not self-indulgent, self-pitying, or a sign of weakness; rather, like Karan's confessions project, it makes it more possible to attend to what's really important.

SELF-COMPASSION

Self-compassion—active cultivation of kindness toward oneself[19]—is one antidote to the unforgiving, harsh, and isolating culture of medicine that becomes manifest in the face of bad outcomes. Practicing self-compassion means neither avoiding negative thoughts nor overidentifying with them. You don't try to confront, overcome, or push through emotional pain, nor do you succumb to it. Rather, you inquire deeply and respond with kindness, clarity, and resolve rather than blame, shame, or despair.

As sensible as self-compassion sounds, doctors have a hard time with the idea. It sounds like self-pity or self-indulgence. But it's none of these—self-compassion means not getting carried away with one's own emotional drama; you don't try to buoy a deflated ego or inflate your self-esteem. Rather, it is a movement toward a healthy balance. People who are able to be more self-compassionate—by either virtue of their prior life experiences or specific training in self-compassion—report feeling better able to own up to their failures and shortcomings without being consumed and paralyzed by negative emotions.[20] They accept their own role in negative events;

they experience a sense of loss and tragedy, yet they don't ruminate obsessively. Self-compassion is ultimately altruistic; it frees you to attend to patients and set aside your own distress. While this is a good lesson for life in general, it's especially important for physicians, who tend to be particularly demanding and unforgiving of themselves.

Marc Lesser is a Zen priest, business consultant, and developer of mindfulness training programs for Fortune 500 companies. Marc would say that self-compassion means knowing yourself and forgetting yourself.[21] Knowing yourself seems self-evident; it helps you find your way in the world. But in a quintessentially paradoxical way, Zen also instructs you to forget yourself. By that, Marc means letting go of rigid assumptions about who you are and recognizing that the assemblage of ideas, habits, and perspectives that you call "me" is more evanescent than you think. Forgetting oneself means abandoning the kinds of self-torture that clinicians habitually engage in when things go wrong. For clinicians—and for anyone else—simultaneously knowing yourself and forgetting yourself helps you respond to error, grief, and loss in a healthier and kinder way.

THINKING BIGGER

Secondary trauma is not unique to anesthesiologists or oncologists or family physicians—all clinicians, regardless of specialty, can be "second victims." The health care system has been slow to respond to this form of clinician distress; few clinicians can honestly say that they work within a culture of awareness, listening, compassion, and support.

But some institutions show signs of hope. The University of Missouri Medical Center has a Second Victim Rapid Response Team, which can be called by clinicians who are feeling distressed. The team offers brief peer and collegial support (Level 1), one-on-one counseling and mentoring by trained peer counselors (Level 2), and referral to mental health professionals for those who are more severely distressed (Level 3).[22] Harvard's Brigham and Women's Hospital offers a peer coaching and support program for distressed physicians. The director, Jo Shapiro, is a surgeon who has trained peer coaches—fellow physicians—to attend to their colleagues in distress.[23] Physicians either refer themselves or refer colleagues who they feel might benefit from one-on-one counseling and coaching. There are few data, making it hard to know how well these efforts work. Yet they represent small steps in the direction toward a culture of caring and support, recognizing that clinician well-being is a sign of health of the health care system overall.

San Francisco is mounting one of the largest efforts to address secondary trauma. San Francisco has enormous social and economic disparities. Their public health clinics care for the most challenging patients—those whose lives are an essay in tragedy, loss, and abandonment and who have repeatedly been failed by the social programs that were intended to help them. The emotional toll on health care workers is large, and attrition and burnout are real problems. Recognizing this, the San Francisco County Health Department instituted a mandatory program in trauma awareness to promote changes in the culture of the health care system as a whole. It's a culture change toward mindful awareness, not just a Band-Aid. Eventually all of San Francisco's nine thousand workers will be trained, and two-thirds of those who have participated so far are working toward concrete changes in their work settings.[24] This kind of coordinated, multilevel intervention is rare in health care organizations and has great promise for sustained change. I'll discuss more about individual and organizational efforts to address burnout and trauma in chapters 10 and 12.

10

Healing the Healer

These are the duties of a physician: First . . . to heal his mind and to give help to himself before giving it to anyone else.

—Epitaph of an Athenian doctor, AD 2[1]

Diane, a midcareer primary care physician, came to our year-long program in mindful practice. She was passionate about clinical care and knew that clinical practice could be deeply fulfilling. However, she was burned out, as she said, "running on empty." Something had to change.

By all accounts, Diane was an exemplary family physician and had excellent clinical judgment. She was a good listener, warm, and empathic, and she won the trust of her patients. Diane would go the extra mile, making home visits for patients who were terminally ill; she'd even drive an elderly patient home at the end of the day to avoid having the patient wait outside in the cold for a city bus. She took care of more than her share of challenging patients and wouldn't turn anyone away. But her dedication took a toll. She was always behind and couldn't spend the time she wanted to with patients.

Meanwhile the landscape of clinical care was changing. More and more, she had to fight with insurance companies so that her patients could get the care that they needed. She had to keep up with eight different prescribing formularies—one for each insurance company—and the rules changed frequently, resulting in prescriptions being denied, and each denial prompted phone calls and paperwork, which cut into face-to-face time with patients. It was, as she put it, sucking her dry.

Then a large health care system bought her practice. Although the health system talked about "quality metrics," in reality these nods to quality amounted to little more than completing meaningless check-boxes[2] and were paled by the pressure to see more patients in less time. "Productivity," not better care. The new electronic health record system provided easy access to patient information, yet because the system was designed primarily to maximize billing, entering clinically relevant data was clumsy and time-consuming. Diane spent more time looking at the computer screen, so much so that on one occasion she didn't notice when a patient left to go to the bathroom and she started talking as if the patient were there. Electronic documentation added an hour to her day, and the promise of increased efficiency was never realized.

This only increased her resolve to work harder to maintain what quality she could. She achieved her productivity goals and quality metrics, but the effort came at a huge cost. At the end of the day, she was beyond tired. She was also increasingly isolated. Like most of her primary care colleagues, Diane had given up hospital privileges because the productivity demands of outpatient practice made it impossible to continue. She barely had time to exchange words with her practice partners during the workday and no longer knew the specialists to whom she referred patients.

The last straw was an encounter with her practice administrator. She saw a patient with worsening depression, and when the "billing specialist" reviewed her documentation of the visit, she suggested that Diane "correct" her diagnosis. Diane had documented the diagnosis as "depression." The administrator suggested that she might write "fatigue" instead. The reason? Money. Reimbursement for mental health diagnoses was just half of that for physical symptoms. While fatigue is part of depression, it's not as accurate a diagnosis. Diane complied. Then she felt nauseous. She realized that her decision was not morally neutral; her limited attention had migrated from the patient's best interest to the financial bottom line.[3]

For the first time in her fifteen-year career as a physician, Diane began to think of her day in terms of quotas and numbers and realized that she was paying less attention to the details of her patients' lives. The bloodless language of health economists had infected her communication patterns and eventually her medical decisions. She felt out of control—of the pace of clinical practice, over hiring employees, or even the design of the office, down to the art on the walls. She began to wonder if medicine was really for her.

Diane took a two-week vacation with her family and felt refreshed, back to her warm and vibrant self. On returning, her symptoms of burnout recurred within days. She couldn't seem to get enough sleep. She had little energy for family and friends. Her staff noticed that she was more irritable, as did her family. Even her patients asked the nurses—or Diane herself—if something was wrong. They knew something had changed, and it wasn't for the better. Diane considered moving to a different practice, but nearly all of the primary care practices in town had already been bought by large health care systems, and her children were in school so a move to a different city would be disruptive. She felt stuck. She thought about quitting practice altogether.

"AN EROSION OF THE SOUL"

Diane's story is, unfortunately, common. It strikes close to home for many doctors. She was a casualty of a national epidemic of physician burnout. After twenty years of research documenting the epidemic, finally in 2016 Dr. Vivek Murthy, the United States surgeon general, announced that physician burnout would be one of two urgent health care problems that the nation needed to address. The reason was obvious—burned-out physicians cannot possibly provide the best care.

The statistics are daunting. Fifty-four percent of physicians nationally reported burnout in 2014, up from 45 percent in 2011.

Those most affected were on the front lines of clinical care—primary care, emergency medicine, and general surgery.[4] Nurses and other health professionals, medical assistants, and secretaries are feeling it too.[5] Although anyone in a high-stress job can experience burnout, in medicine it is particularly nefarious, and patients have reason to worry. Burned-out physicians are more likely to take shortcuts, make diagnostic errors, and prescribe recklessly.[6] They order too many tests and refer more, just because it takes too much effort to think through problems themselves.[7] They don't communicate well, with their patients[8] or their colleagues, and are more likely to abuse alcohol and drugs and engage in unprofessional behaviors— shady billing practices, providing narcotics to addicts, inappropriate use of social media, and violating patient confidentiality. Some physicians are jumping ship. Of primary care internal-medicine physicians starting practice, a quarter of them will quit within five years,[9] and others are taking early retirement. Replacing them is costly—over $300,000 per physician.[10]

Not everyone catches burnout in time. The majority of burned-out physicians will still be burned out a year later. A colleague, an excellent family physician whom I'd mentored when she was a resident, recently took an early retirement. The new medical records system—the four thousand clicks a day and completing charts at midnight—did her in.[11] My own primary care doctor retired last year after I had been a patient of his for only two years. When he left, the practice sent a terse and impersonal letter that said that he was closing his practice after thirty years to "teach and mentor." When I started with him after my previous primary care doctor left practice, he said that he would be good for another five to ten years. It's not difficult to guess what was behind his decision. I called his office to get a personal recommendation for a new physician. I was directed to a list of three hundred local primary care doctors, only eight of whom were taking new patients, all of whom had just finished training. I felt abandoned. Clearly, something had changed.

Dr. Christina Maslach, a psychologist who has devoted her career to studying burnout, describes it as "an erosion of the soul."[12]

Across all human services professions, Maslach found that burnout consisted of three factors: emotional exhaustion, depersonalization (treating people as objects), and a feeling of low personal accomplishment. This three-headed monster makes work an intolerable burden rather than a source of purpose and meaning, making physicians either work harder and harder or just give up.

Medical practice has always been intense. To give you a sense of the emotional burden of practice, let me take you through a typical four-hour session in my primary care office. I saw eleven patients. First was a thirty-eight-year-old amputee, blind and on dialysis due to diabetes, who was about to have his other leg amputated. The next patient, recently inherited from a now-retired physician, was addicted to prescription narcotics and fell asleep at the wheel, plowing into the car in front of him, shattering his knee and his shoulder. He had consumed an entire week's worth of oxycodone in two days, and now he wanted more. Later in the morning were the struggling parents bringing their violent and hyperactive child, who was recently returned to them from foster care. Then, a fifty-five-year-old man with AIDS who forgot to get his blood tests and didn't go for the X-ray to evaluate his pneumonia; I realized that he had the beginnings of AIDS dementia and had no family to care for him. The day ended with the repeated denials of a brilliant psychotherapist whose liver was being consumed by alcoholic cirrhosis. Without the inner scaffolding of presence and mental stability and the outer scaffolding of collegial and institutional support, no one can be expected to respond humanely to all this tragedy.

But now, in the age of the corporatization and widgetization of medicine, there is a new kind of burnout, a slow, relentless "deterioration of values, dignity, spirit and will"[13] that comes from the structure of health care itself. Patients become "covered lives," and the intimacy of a clinical encounter is reduced to RVUs—relative value units—the productivity metrics that determine how much doctors are paid. The more that doctors' work is tied to computer screens and the more "functionalities" that are added to the electronic health record, the worse burnout becomes. Casualties of efficiency, doctors turn off their emotions. They can't wait until the end of the day, the weekend, retirement. They back their cars into their parking spaces so they can make a quick exit at the end of the day. Patients wonder if their doctors care at all.

Burned-out physicians are not only alienated from patients; they are also alienated from themselves. They feel as if they are on an assembly line, and the opportunity for the rich and rewarding human interactions they imagined when they chose to be doctors is reduced to a mere transaction of information. Recently I reviewed an emergency room chart for a six-month-old patient of mine who had had a fever. Apparently, the electronic health record required that the physician fill in templates about smoking, alcohol consumption, and sexual risk behaviors. The amazing thing is that the physician actually wasted his time by checking the boxes. With enough of these occurrences, feeling battered by systems they cannot change, some doctors capitulate and go numb and only later come to a crushing realization that they have abandoned their values. Others feel that their impact is nil, become depressed, and think only about escape. In one study, 17 percent of those reporting burnout considered suicide in the previous year.[14] This is frightening, given that doctors kill themselves at a rate higher than those in any other profession. I've personally known several.

The problem is not only overwork; it's crisis of meaning, resilience, and community. The toxic combination of high responsibility, low sense of control, and isolation sets the stage for a sense of exhaustion, powerlessness, and helplessness.[15] The stresses due to a dysfunctional health care system and the culture of medicine are real, and the health care community has an obligation to fix them. Putting clinicians in morally compromising situations, installing electronic health record systems that are sculpted around billing rather than good patient care, and placing increasing pressure on clinicians to see more patients without regard to quality are practices that need to change.

THE INNER ENVIRONMENT

But changing the health care system won't solve it all. It is important to recognize that burnout has affected clinicians for centuries, and important causes of burnout reside within clinicians themselves. For the first time in memory, perhaps precipitated by the perfect storm of the heavy burden of suffering in the clinic and the increasing dysfunction of the health care system, some doctors are finally paying attention to their inner environment in a systematic way and finding ways to bring greater presence and resilience to the practice of medicine.

Imagine you're choosing a doctor or that you're hiring a physician to join a practice. What qualities would you want the doctor to have? When I ask this question of the general public or groups of clinicians—no matter what their profession or specialty—the answers are always the same. They want someone who is altruistic and hardworking, has excellent technical skills, is knowledgeable, has good judgment, is empathic and caring, and has equanimity in the face of tragedy and loss.

Yet, even these very *desirable* personality characteristics make doctors psychologically vulnerable.[16] Those who are detail oriented can become compulsive, subjecting patients to too many tests and procedures "just to be sure" and waking at night because they think that they may have forgotten something.[17] Altruistic, service-oriented doctors tend to overcommit and then get exhausted trying to follow through. Truly skilled doctors might believe that they can do it all—feeling omniscient, omnipotent, and unable to admit mistakes—a dangerous combination in medicine. Or they feel insecure. When physicians are asked if they ever feel like an impostor, a remarkable percentage (up to 43 percent) say yes.[18] Of all personality factors, the most closely associated with burnout is rigidity. When unaware of his rigidity, a doctor might insist that his is the single best approach for each problem, and blame his frustration and ineffectiveness on other people (including patients) rather than looking inside himself.[19] Even being empathic takes its toll when doctors don't recognize their secondary trauma and negative emotions.[20] Disturbingly, some clinicians wear stress and burnout as badges of honor, part of the macho culture of medicine that further compounds the anguish and isolation of distressed clinicians.[21] Too often, self-awareness is lacking.

WHY SOME PEOPLE DON'T BURN OUT

Things don't have to be this way. Some clinicians, albeit stressed, fare better than others. They not only cope and adapt, they grow in response to challenges so that the next challenge becomes more tractable. In fact, the right kinds and the right amounts of stress can make us stronger—"stress inoculation." Bones and muscles and brains and hearts grow stronger—more resilient—when you exercise and stress them in the right ways. Bearing weight strengthens bones; without stress, they weaken and crumble. Muscles, too, need exercise or else they atrophy. We thrive on mental challenges, and without them we become dull. Resilience is, in Nicholas Taleb's words, becoming "antifragile."[22] We develop resilience best when we are at our growing edge—just a hair beyond our capacities.

We often think about resilience as the capacity to get through a hard time. However, in high-stress professions, the pressures are ongoing and crises are unpredictable; real resilience is being prepared to be unprepared. Only in the past thirty years have psychologists focused on understanding resilience as a positive attribute and not merely a reaction to trauma. However, much of what we know about resilience is from studies of animals in laboratory environments and people who have endured interpersonal violence, a debilitating injury, war, torture, or natural disasters, not those who have voluntarily chosen a lifetime of work that they knew would be emotionally demanding.

Psychiatrists Steve Southwick and Dennis Charney interviewed former POWs, Special Forces instructors, and civilians who had experienced severe psychological traumas such as rape, sexual abuse, the loss of a limb, or cancer.[23] They found that in spite of these extreme events, remarkably few developed depression or post-traumatic stress disorder.[24] Southwick and Charney identified ten "resilience factors" that would make sense to most of us: realistic optimism, facing fear, moral compass, religion and spirituality, social support, role models, physical fitness, brain fitness, cognitive and emotional flexibility, and a sense of meaning and purpose. Personality is important too. Just as some personality factors are associated with greater risks of burnout, others confer greater resilience. Psychologists Richard Ryan and Edward Deci point to three qualities: the ability to form warm and caring relationships with others — so-called secure attachment — a sense of personal autonomy, and perceiving oneself as competent and up to the task.[25]

Resilience is mirrored in our biochemical and genetic makeup. Those who thrive despite severe trauma are biochemically different from their less resilient peers. They have lower levels of stress hormones and neuropeptide Y, the "anxiety" neurotransmitter. They have higher levels of serotonin, which is associated with positive mood, and higher levels of dopamine in the reward centers of their brains. They have higher levels of "brain-derived neurotropic factor," which directs the brain to grow new neural pathways.[26] Because resilience seems to be affected by caring and trusting human relationships, most likely oxytocin — the hormone associated with love and affiliation — is also involved. It appears that not only do resilient people trigger the release of higher levels of these neurotransmitters and hormones, but they also have more receptors for them. Signals are more easily transmitted. And sometimes the receptors are of a different subtype altogether to which a neurotransmitter binds more avidly.

We are now just learning what might lead the body to produce more of these substances and to place more — and more avid — receptors on nerve cells. Just as I discussed in chapter 3, it's epigenetic regulation; social epigenetics to be more precise. Genes that encode for neurotransmitters and receptors turn on when you're in a supportive and safe environment and turn off when you feel vulnerable and traumatized. Those experiencing secondary trauma, isolation, and lack of support are literally—on a biochemical level—less able to muster the resilience they need. This means that doctors who aren't allowed time to debrief after a patient death or who submit to meaningless bureaucratic tasks are likely to become less and less resilient. Admittedly, resilience (and gene regulation) is to some extent influenced by past events which cannot be changed, such as prenatal influences and early childhood traumas. But it is tantalizing to consider recent research by psychologist Douglas Johnson at the Naval Health Research Center in San Diego; his research group demonstrated the mindfulness programs for military recruits promoted self-awareness and resilience and, in doing so, enhanced their "healthy" gene expression.[27]

TIPPY AND UNFLIPPABLE

How do people become more resilient? Part of the answer has to do with mental stability. I am not an expert kayaker, but I do enjoy it. A few years ago, I bought a kayak. In the store, the salesperson talked about primary instability and secondary instability. At first, I was confused. Why would I want to buy a kayak that was unstable? He explained. Kayaks with primary instability are more maneuverable, and it takes less effort to guide them around rocks, sharp bends, and standing waves in a river, but they also feel tippier. Secondary instability refers to how easily the kayak will capsize. Because I wanted a boat that was responsive and I had no interest in getting wet when I least expected it, I chose a kayak that had quite a bit of primary instability and a fair degree of secondary stability.

Once I had it in the water, it took some getting used to. It felt really tippy. It took me a while to distinguish primary from secondary instability and to have the confidence that the kayak wouldn't flip over. With time, I came to tolerate feeling "unbalanced" and I could maneuver the kayak more effortlessly, and I realized that fighting the primary instability put me at greater risk than using it to my advantage. I even came to relish the tippiness. I realized that

I had made progress when one day, kayaking across a lake with a strong crosswind, I leaned into the wind, so much so that I was at a thirty-degree angle, water coming way up one side of the kayak. I was moving in a straight line and the kayak didn't flip.

Mental stability works the same way. It's a dynamic equilibrium. You're never completely in balance. Just as I enjoy the tippiness of my kayak, I've come to enjoy the unpredictable and chaotic corners of medicine; the next patient could be a day old or one hundred years old, and the patient's issues could be trivial or life threatening. There's a certain off-balance thrill to navigating unexpected twists with aplomb.

REMINDERS

In difficult times, I keep coming back to three important "reminders" about resilience. The first is that *resilience is a capacity that can be grown.*[28] With training, you can gain more control over your behavior and well-being, relate to stress in healthier ways, and feel differently about yourself. Resilience doesn't mean hardening the heart; quite the opposite, resilience is about adopting lightness, a sense of humor, and flexibility. You change your personality, just a bit, becoming more focused, more tippable, and less flippable. Participants in our year-long mindful practice program did just that. Over time, they scored higher on two of the Big Five personality factors that relate to focused attention and mental stability—and the changes endured.[29] While the party line in personality psychology had been that personality was immutable after age thirty, more recently researchers have studied people whose personalities *had* changed throughout their lifetimes. Those who changed had three qualities: they were adept at observing themselves, observing others, and listening attentively.[30] In short, they were mindful.

The second reminder is that *well-being is about engagement, not withdrawal.* This is not intuitive. If a situation is pleasant, it makes sense to stick around and want more. But what if a situation is unpleasant? It's only natural to want to get away and avoid people you find difficult. While these survival strategies might help in the short run, the same old problems and their maladaptive solutions are still there. Preventing burnout and developing resilience have more to do with presence than escape.

The third reminder is that *mindfulness is a community activity*. When I was in Bhutan a few years ago, I walked past hermitages scattered high above tiny Himalayan villages in some of the most isolated spots in the world, in caves and steep ravines, beside glaciers and atop three-thousand-foot cliffs. The monks doing three-year-long solitary retreats might not even see the villagers who would bring them food each week, yet they could do what they were doing *because* of the knowledge that the villagers were supporting their efforts and that other monks in other hermitages were engaged in a similar effort. Even in isolation they felt—and were—part of a community.

The same is true for the rest of us; we need a sense of community to sustain a mindful vision. Yet, over the past few years, hospital doctors' lounges have closed, personal relationships among clinicians have eroded, and in the outpatient setting clinicians know each other only as faceless characters sharing an electronic chart. Creating community requires visionary leadership, yet this vision and the leaders to promote it are lacking in the current health care environment.

WHAT IS WELL-BEING, ANYWAY?

I bristle when people say that the key to well-being is achieving "work-life balance." Those who see "life" as everything outside work, necessitating "balance," implicitly assume that when you're at work, you're not fully alive, a sad state of affairs for those of us who are in a profession that is capable of providing such deep rewards (and that takes up so much of our waking existence).[31] It reflects a deeper problem, though. By placing the blame for your unhappiness exclusively on things external to yourself (the work environment), you're assuming that by containing work—by compartmentalizing, pushing it away, or making it "not-me"—you might be happier. This is a trap.

Marc Lesser recounts a famous Zen dialogue:[32]

The monk arrives at the monastery and says to the teacher, "I've arrived. Please give me your teaching."

The teacher says, "Have you eaten your breakfast?"

The monk responds, "Yes, I have."

The teacher says, "Wash your bowl."

The monk understood. What could be more obvious?

Marc explains that this indirect and somewhat bizarre answer is intended to free the mind from habitual and monocular views of a situation and instead invite you to look at your current experience, right here, right now. Marc comments, "If you were to ask, 'How can I find work-life balance?,' I might be inclined to ask if you have eaten your breakfast. . . . And, assuming you have, I suggest you wash your bowl."

Marc continues:

Attempting to achieve work-life balance, as though something is missing or something is wrong (either with you or with your situation), is a set-up for failure, for stress, and for anything but balance. Instead, experiment by bringing your attention to the activities that make up your work. Notice the activities and notice your inner dialogue, the stories you weave, as well as your feelings. Just this act of paying attention can produce positive change—a bit of slowing down, a little more space—opening up the possibility of change, of more calm, even of more appreciation.

Marc's answer invites a deeper and more important question: What is well-being, anyway? We know that when people have a deep sense of meaning and fulfillment, the more superficial trappings—what you have in terms of achievement or pleasure—are less important and may even get you off track. We can tolerate long hours and even welcome stress if work intrinsically brings a sense of purpose, satisfaction, joy, and meaning. That deeper kind of well-being, one that's worth achieving, is what Aristotle called *eudaimonia*. *Eudaimonia* is true human flourishing; it *results from* and *leads to* being more fully engaged with one's work in a healthy and positive way[33] while recognizing that the world is messy, chaotic, imperfect, and not always pleasant. Pushing away only makes matters worse.

THE 20 PERCENT RULE

My wife, Deborah, tells a story about Mary Pedersen, her extraordinary and somewhat eccentric seventh-grade teacher. Deb was thirteen years old and living in Denmark for a year. Mary asked Deb, "Honeylamb"—she really did say this!—"honeylamb, what do *you* like? What do you *like*?" Deb was thunderstruck. No one had ever asked her that question. It got her thinking and led her first to writing, then to Renaissance history, then to seventeenth-century music. Fifteen years later, we visited Mary in Denmark (and she called me "honeylamb" too) in her cottage so overgrown with vines and rosebushes that the patio was reduced to an area just large enough for three small chairs. We learned that she had been a Shakespearean actor; in her youth, she left a secure academic path in England to join a theater troupe. While on tour in Denmark, she fell in love and found a job there at an English-speaking school. Although she worked as an artist, an actor, and a teacher until she was seventy, she felt that she never "worked" a day in her life. We should all be as fortunate as Mary Pedersen. Her capacity for joy was infectious, and Deb caught the bug. She too feels that her career as a musician isn't "work" in the way that most of us think about it, in part because of Mary's influence.

Not many of us have had teachers like Mary who remind us to stop and think, "What, in my work setting, gives me the greatest sense of joy, fulfillment, and meaning?" Think about that question for a moment and then consider—here's the clincher—"In a typical week, how much of my time do I actually spend doing those activities?" It doesn't have to be 100 percent; few people are that fortunate. Research shows that if physicians spend even 20 percent of their work time in the activities that they regard as the most meaningful, they're much less likely to be burned out, meaning that they're more able to tolerate the difficult moments.[34] Makes sense, but most doctors—and others who have some control over their work lives—have never asked themselves these fundamental questions. People shouldn't wait until they are feeling burned out to reflect on what's most nourishing about their work.

THE EARLY SIGNS

Physicians know that it's easier to manage any illness during the early stages rather than waiting until it is full-blown. They know the long list of late signs of distress—insomnia, depression, chronic pain, migraines, GI symptoms, drinking too much, relationship problems, and more. They know that early signs are harder to detect, so it takes vigilance. Yet ironically, doctors are particularly at risk for not seeing these early signs because doctors tend to be stoical. They think that stress is a normal part of the job, are notorious for delaying seeking care, and for self-medicating.

An honest self-appraisal is the first step. During workshops, I'll ask participants to rate their burnout using Maslach's burnout scale,[35] or the simple diagram on the next page. You'll see a list of attributes of burnout and well-being and a scale of 1 to 10. Try it. Are you a 1, a 5, or a 10? As you're doing this, stop, think, and feel the impact of your work environment on your life. Perhaps this might be the moment when you can no longer underestimate your distress.

With training, you can bring these warning signs to your awareness before they get out of hand. Training starts with noticing. Ask yourself, *What are some of my early warning signs of distress in the workplace setting?* Start with the body. *What bodily sensations and behaviors do I notice?* Most of the time, we feel these early warnings as bodily sensations—a tightness in the shoulders, a knot in

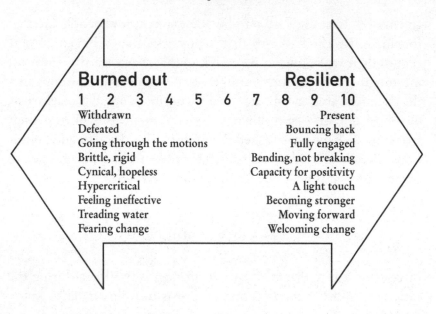

Burned out								Resilient	
1	2	3	4	5	6	7	8	9	10

Burned out	Resilient
Withdrawn	Present
Defeated	Bouncing back
Going through the motions	Fully engaged
Brittle, rigid	Bending, not breaking
Cynical, hopeless	Capacity for positivity
Hypercritical	A light touch
Feeling ineffective	Becoming stronger
Treading water	Moving forward
Fearing change	Welcoming change

the stomach, shakiness. *Next, explore any emotions that accompany those warning signs: What are they?* The emotions that often accompany the bodily sensations might be feelings of impatience, fear or anger, and sometimes just a sense of disconnection and blandness. *Now, be aware of thoughts, ideas, interpretations, and judgments that accompany these warning signs.* Sensations and emotions may be accompanied by specific thoughts—such as thinking that you're feeling inadequate in some way. You might notice that your behavior is different—you drive faster, eat less, put off important tasks, clean your desk, or buy things you don't really need—before you consciously register that you are tired, stressed, or annoyed.

One early warning sign for me is when I start making more typos than usual. It's annoying. I go back and correct the error, then compensate by typing faster. Then I pound harder on the keys, as if I could beat them into submission. It only gets worse. I get angry at the computer (*Why is the spell-checker in the medical record so clunky?*), then the clinic (*Why did they have to schedule three extra patients for me today?*), and finally patients themselves (*Why does she always come with forty complaints to deal with in a twenty-minute visit?*).

Awareness of these early warning signs can provide a window into our inner state before things get unmanageable. I call them "friends"; they are protectors and reminders. When I notice my typing deteriorating, I can stop for a moment and appreciate that I have a choice, a choice I had not previously acknowledged: I can choose to get annoyed at myself and pound harder, or I can summon a state of curiosity, saying to myself, "Oh, here I am making typos. I wonder what that's about. Am I feeling rushed? Is the task unpleasant? Do I need to feel that way? Is it useful to respond in this way? Can I do anything about it?" It may seem easy to take a new perspective, yet too often all of us just let the pressures mount. Because most of us don't have habits that constantly put us in touch with the early warning signs of stress, we have to develop them. It takes intention, practice, and discipline—qualities that doctors and most high-functioning professionals often bring to other domains of their lives.

When being mindful, I am aware of how my expectations and emotions condition what I see and that I can take a new perspective or readjust the lens through which I see the world. I engage in metacognition: thinking about and appraising my thinking and emotions. It's saying to myself, "I'm feeling pretty stressed. What's that about?" Then asking myself, "Is this situation really altogether negative?" And "Is there something I can learn from it?" I realize that my original view may have been biased or myopic. I recalibrate. Research suggests that those who are able to recalibrate and take a new perspective may grow new neural connections in brain structures associated with emotional intelligence and emotion regulation.[36]

RESILIENCE TRAINING

Some of the most interesting research on resilience training comes from military settings, with soldiers who were about to be deployed into war zones. I initially had trouble with research about people who were being trained to control and kill—and not to empower

Ronald Epstein, M.D.

and heal—until I realized that I was making assumptions that might not be quite true. In many ways, medical settings resemble military settings. In both health care and the military, the physical and emotional stresses are ongoing and extreme, and the training is rigorous and all-consuming. In both settings, the dictum is "first do no harm" (although I wish that doctors and generals would keep that in mind more often) and not be trigger-happy (medications and surgery can kill as well as heal). In both settings, problems are complex. You need mental stability, effective communication, ethical conduct, and wisdom to manage unexpected situations rarely encountered in civilian life. Both settings have hierarchies that often do more harm than good, bringing a huge risk of disconnection between those who are in charge and those who are on the front lines. Both soldiers and doctors experience vicarious trauma frequently—they witness the unbearable suffering, loss, grief, dismemberment, disintegration, and destruction of people who deserve better. Both professions involve huge personal sacrifices, and reflection and self-awareness are not part of either professional culture.

Military mind-fitness programs with a strong emphasis on meditation practice have had positive effects.[37] Participants recovered more rapidly after stressful events. Their heart rates and breathing and stress hormone levels normalized sooner, and they experienced fewer ill effects from subsequent stresses. They made better decisions, had fewer lapses in attention, and were better able to tolerate adversity.

To address the controversy that such programs might just make more attentive—but heartless—killers, the developers of the program have a counterargument: reducing emotional reactivity can reduce the reckless or unethical behaviors that only compound the tragedy of war. They claim that by improving emotional intelligence, soldiers might work as a team and win the hearts and minds of others. I hope that is true. I raise this controversial parallel to medical practice because these studies point to ways in which health professionals and others doing "combat duty" in the public service can become more mindful.

RECAPTURING PURPOSE AND MEANING

Whenever I see a distressed clinician learn to be more resilient, I wonder how she did it. The health care environment has only gotten worse, with more administrative burdens and less social support. The first hurdle is awareness. Diane knew she was distressed, as do most participants in our workshops. They've seen the warning signs. Over the course of a year, Diane started a regular meditation practice, just ten to fifteen minutes each morning, and used an app for her smartphone that would remind her and time her sessions. More important, she prompted herself to incorporate mindful moments into her day—a habit of pausing, opening, relaxing—rather than just plowing through. Even brief moments of self-care were powerful reminders to focus more on what was truly important. She adopted a practice of gratitude, each day intentionally naming one thing for which she was grateful; it helped her to recalibrate. Gradually she saw more clearly which external factors she couldn't change—completing meaningless checklists, wrestling with insurance companies, and dealing with unwieldy electronic record systems—and her attitude changed. She learned that she didn't have to respond to every request made by patients, administrators, and insurance companies, and she mastered a few more shortcuts so that she could work with the electronic health record system more effectively. She started a small insurrection in her office—she put *her* photographs on the walls, and others did the same. She realized that the computer screen could be a barrier, so she had the computer screen remounted and rearranged her office so that she and the patient could look at the screen together—it improved communication and helped her to feel more connected with patients, even when she had to type or look something up. These small changes reflected an incremental change of focus and attitude. She was more honest with herself, listened more deeply to patients and colleagues, and felt a greater sense of community. Despite kayaking in rough waters, she felt that she was no longer about to drown.

11

Becoming Mindful

When you practice being mindful, you reshape your brain. Every year, hundreds of scientific articles explore how this happens and under what conditions. But the very idea that the adult brain could be reshaped was radical until thirty years ago; psychologists and neuroscientists had underestimated the human capacity for neuroplasticity—how our brains continue to grow and develop throughout life. The good news is that you can do more than keep your brain from withering; you can make new connections among neurons and help to grow your brain.

Some of the earliest work on neuroplasticity was done with London taxi drivers. I drove a taxicab in Manhattan while taking my premed courses at Columbia, so I was familiar with the rigors of the job and the creative approaches drivers employ to navigate complex cities. But London is much more complicated than New York, and the training to become a taxi driver is much more rigorous. Potential drivers need to learn the 320 "best routes" connecting thousands of "places of note" along the sixty thousand roads within a six-mile radius of central London—almost none of which go in a straight line and many of which are one-way and change names several times. The exams to become a taxi driver in London (known as Appearances) are notoriously difficult, and people typically spend three to four years acquiring "the Knowledge," a deep familiarity with the particulars of the roads and places of note and how the routes that connect them must be combined and altered, depending on traffic conditions, to get to each destination efficiently.

Eleanor Maguire and Katherine Woollett, neuropsychologists at University College London, were curious. They wanted to see if changes could be noted in the brains of the taxi drivers, particularly in the posterior hippocampus—the area of the brain concerned with spatial memory. They scanned the brains of seventeen taxi drivers and eighteen bus drivers. They found that the posterior hippocampus was larger in taxi drivers, who need to constantly find new routes, compared with bus drivers, who don't.[1] The more the taxi drivers drove, the larger the posterior hippocampus. Then Maguire and Woollett studied seventy-nine taxi trainees and thirty-nine controls. Each driver had psychological testing and MRI scans at the start and end of their training. In those who passed the exam, the posterior hippocampus had grown. It hadn't in the controls or in those who failed.[2] Of note, those who did well spent twice as much time studying as those who didn't.

The ability to assimilate vast quantities of knowledge and construct mental maps would sound familiar to any medical student. Medical students learn thousands of new words during their first two years of medical school, and each word—and the concept that it represents—is linked to other words in complex ways. Just as taxi drivers create mental maps of cities, medical students create mental maps of physiological and pathological pathways that manifest as health and disease. With repeated firing, these neural connections become better "lubricated," so that mental tasks (such as memory and association) that previously took significant effort eventually become automatic. In time, the words are linked to real patients and thereby acquire personal meaning and emotional valence. The brain grows new connections—it rewires and reshapes itself. While behavioral scientist Donald Hebb proposed, as early as 1949, that "neurons that fire together wire together,"[3] until recently you couldn't actually see the rewiring in action. Now with sophisticated neuroimaging, it is possible to see how, with increasing practice, parts of the brain actually grow. The brain grows not only when you practice memory tasks and motor skills, but also when you practice "meta-skills"—skills of being attentive, curious, openminded, and present. Admittedly, while the psychological and physical benefits of developing attentiveness and other aspects of mindfulness are clear, our knowledge of the actual changes in brain structure, chemistry, and functioning is still rudimentary.

WHAT MAKES A GREAT DOCTOR?

By the time they are a few years out from completing training, master clinicians have shaped their brains in particular ways to enhance specific abilities depending on what their work requires—knowledge, good judgment, emotional responsiveness, compassion, and technical skill. But how do master clinicians get that way? How can we help more clinicians get there?

The answers come from reexamining what we mean by expertise. In psychology, education, and health care, researchers have struggled with the question of expertise. For a long time researchers thought that natural talent accounted for a lot of it; you had a particular aptitude for singing or science, or soccer.

Psychologist Karl Anders Ericsson took another view—that expertise is largely a product of experience. Ericsson observed chess masters, musicians, and athletes and found that true masters don't get that way just because they have natural talent; they engage in what he calls "deliberate practice."[4] Remember that the taxi drivers who passed the test had studied twice as much as those who didn't. In Ericsson's estimation, it takes about ten thousand hours of practice, or ten years, to have expertise in complex skills, whether the skills are chess playing or brain surgery (or taxi driving). However, it has to be high-quality practice, with supervision and feedback.

Ericsson also explored how doctors become experts, noting that expertise is different in medicine than in other pursuits. Chess players, musicians, and athletes typically start acquiring their skills as children, whereas doctors typically begin to acquire their skills when they're in their twenties. Musicians, chess players, and athletes learn how emotions and attitudes affect performance—there's the "inner game" and the "outer game." There is much less talk of emotions in medical training. In chess, music, and sports, it's usually clear that when things go wrong it's due to someone having made an error. In medicine it's not so clear. A patient's outcome is not completely attributable to a doctor's skill; so much depends on the particulars of each patient that are out of a physician's control. Most important, for musicians, training is much more intimate and involves direct observation, critique, and feedback. When I was studying music, I'd be one-on-one with my piano teacher for an hour every week. Over time I'd anticipate and internalize what my teacher might say, and gradually I was able to critique myself. While surgeons benefit from direct supervision in the operating room, in most branches of medicine it is very different. When I was a medical student and a resident, I'd tell my supervising physicians what I had seen and accomplished, but only rarely did they actually observe me with a patient. My mentor George Engel suggested that we imagine what would happen if piano lessons were that way—you'd just report to your teacher what you had done well and where you perceived there were problems.[5] You certainly wouldn't get to Carnegie Hall that way.

Brothers Stuart and Hubert Dreyfus at the University of California, Berkeley, also observed professionals in a variety of fields. They developed a model in which they described a hierarchy from novice, to competent, proficient, and expert, later adding a level for master.[6] For the Dreyfus brothers, expertise involved making automatic what for novices would be deliberate and effortful. The Dreyfuses suggested that experts could then reserve their cognitive resources for more complex tasks. For example, the nurse who took my blood pressure before a recent visit to my doctor was talking to me throughout. An expert, she could easily divide her attention between the automatic task and the (hopefully more interesting) interpersonal interaction, whereas a nursing student would have had to devote her full attention to what she was hearing through the stethoscope. Because these tasks become so automatic, experts, according to the Dreyfus brothers, often have difficulty describing exactly what they do.

Expertise is not merely automatic, though it also includes the ability to alternate—effortlessly—between automatic and effortful cognitive processing.[7] When a nurse in my dentist's office took my blood pressure two days after I saw my doctor, she was chatting just like the previous nurse. Then, suddenly she stopped. She took my pressure again, this time paying closer attention (I was not looking forward to the dental procedure, and my body let us know it). She slowed down. She noted an unusually high blood pressure. She switched gears.

Not every nurse would. While the ten-thousand-hours formula might work for developing basic skills, only if the practice is mindful will people learn to switch from automatic to effortful, to slow down when they should. Mindless practice, in contrast, leads to being an "experienced non-expert," repeating the same mistakes over and over, without the insight to know why. Conversely, "true experts" are mindful and adaptive; they recognize when something's amiss before others do. They observe and respond to context, then switch gears, slowing down and improvising.[8] It's like jazz.[9]

VOLUNTARILY BRINGING BACK A WANDERING ATTENTION

Cultivating and sustaining attention is the sine qua non of good care. Over 120 years ago, William James devoted one of the first chapters of his *Principles of Psychology* to attention. James described— remarkably accurately—how attention works, setting the stage for future research. But he didn't know how to cultivate it. He said, "The faculty of voluntarily bringing back a wandering attention, over and over again, is the very root of judgment, character, and will. . . . An education which should improve this faculty would be the education par excellence. But it is easier to define this ideal than to give practical directions for bringing it about."[10]

Attention training is now common practice. It takes remarkably little to augment your capacity to attend. Even after a week of meditating thirty minutes a day, executive attention improves—if you recall, executive attention helps to reduce and reconcile conflicts between competing demands on your attention (such as someone talking to you when you're trying to add up a column of numbers).[11] After eight weeks of practice you'd likely have better sustained focus (top-down attention) and you'd be less likely to be derailed by the unimportant. With longer practice, some studies suggest that you'd be able to manage your precious cognitive resources more effectively and switch among mental tasks more quickly. You would be better able to remember key information, even when asked to multitask in highly stressful environments.[12] With practice, you'd be more likely to notice and name your emotions, allowing you to respond more intelligently to strong feelings; you'd feel less frustrated when under high cognitive load; and you'd ruminate less about the past and worry less about the future. You'd become more present and more mentally fit.

If you continued practicing, you'd become more aware of how your mind works. You could more readily identify when you are focused or distracted, when you're being curious and when you're more shut down. You'd become a connoisseur of types and qualities of your states of attending and distraction—just as the Inuit become connoisseurs of snow and sommeliers become connoisseurs of wine.[13] Functional brain imaging might show thickening of the gray matter in the brain, deeper folds of the brain (gyrification), and increased connectivity. Studies done by psychologist Al Kaszniak at the University of Arizona suggest that attention training can reverse the natural decline of cognition with age.[14]

BEGINNING

Zen teachers often tell beginners, "Don't meditate, just pay attention." This is because for some people the word *meditation* carries with it expectations and associations.

Meditation practice is skill building,[15] an education of the mind through first-person inquiry.[16] Some people associate meditation with self-absorption, so to make the purpose clear, I call it attention training, awareness training, compassion training, or, simply, practice. I emphasize that the ultimate purpose of meditation is to reduce suffering in the world, not to feel good about yourself. Debate rages about whether meditation is intrinsically "spiritual," but it depends on how you define "spiritual." If you see "spiritual" as anything that lends meaning and coherence to the world, then perhaps meditation is. It certainly does not require any particular religious or philosophical belief system, other than believing that by knowing yourself better you can be more effective at realizing what is most important.[17]

Most practitioners use two or more practices at different points during their training. It's like exercise—you wouldn't only do push-ups if you wanted to get fit. We are only beginning to understand the way in which each meditation practice develops a different part of the brain, and no one can say whether one particular method is "better" than another; they are just different.[18] In the appendix I describe the two most common and widely studied meditation practices, which are known as focused attention practice and open awareness practice. Briefly, focused attention involves focusing the mind on an "object"—the breath or a mantra. Open awareness is a disciplined practice of being aware of whatever is happening right now, in the present moment, but without attention to any particular object. Other practices, such as body scan and compassion training, were described earlier in the book (see chapters 3 and 8).

But what's the threshold? How much (or how little) attention training do we need? It seems that even small doses can make a difference, at least in the short run. A few people even say that their first experience with meditation was transformative—they feel that a door had been opened and would never again be closed. Those who practice daily become more adept than those who don't. And others notice. I was tantalized by a small pilot study by David Schroeder and his colleagues in Portland, Oregon, in which primary care teams who underwent mindfulness training found that their patient ratings were directly proportional to the amount of time they spent practicing.[19] It's not just quantity, though; quality of practice matters too. Just daydreaming won't get you there.[20]

THE BODY

I've wondered why most contemplative practices start with attention to sensory experiences. Only now, though, are neuroscientists, cognitive scientists, and philosophers converging on an understanding that emotions are fundamentally embodied, inextricably linked to our bodily states.[21] We gnash our teeth when working on a difficult problem or grip our seats during a horror movie. Our language is filled with bodily metaphors: *a pain in the neck*, *heartache*, and *shouldering a burden*. We call informative and helpful intuitions *gut feelings*. We describe people in terms of sensory experience: people who are emotionally distant are *cold* and those who seem close are *warm*. We use kinesthetic and spatial expressions: *feeling down in the dumps* or *up to par*; *on top of things* or *under the weather*. We mentally simulate bodily sensations in order to retrieve memories of events, and during exercises such as the body scan (described in chapter 3), by directing awareness to the body we become more aware of thoughts and emotions.

It works the other way too. We can evoke emotions by assuming different bodily postures and expressions. Standing tall imbues dignity; kneeling and bowing evoke submission. My piano lessons always started with posture. In the military, "attention" is a physical stance, which presumably calls up a certain state of mind. Assuming a dignified sitting posture is the first task for beginner meditation students with the goal of preparing them for awareness, mental stability, and humility.

Francesc Borrell-Carrió, an astute colleague, noticed that doctors smile when they greet a patient, even those that they don't particularly like.[22] He wondered why. In those situations, smiling has nothing to do with being happy. It's about preparing oneself to be hospitable, to be present, to understand, and to help. It inspires an attitude of welcoming and good humor and not clinging too tenuously to any preconceived ideas one might have. Even a forced smile can make a difference in terms of how you understand your own and someone else's emotions. In a psychology experiment, psychologist Arthur Glenberg divided participants into two groups; one group held a pencil between the teeth to engage the smile muscles, whereas the other held a pencil between the upper lip and the nose to engage frown muscles. When engaging the smile muscles, participants processed information about pleasant events more readily than about unpleasant events, whereas the reverse was true if they engaged the frown muscles.[23] Psychologist Al Kaszniak has demonstrated greater activation of the zygomatic ("smile") muscles in long-term meditators, perhaps one contribution to their feeling more positive emotions.[24] Science has taken twenty-five hundred years to catch up, providing experimental evidence for what practitioners have always held as obvious.[25]

INTERPERSONAL MINDFULNESS

I asked a recently retired leader at our hospital about his uncanny ability to handle difficult situations. His days were filled with meetings during which he'd often have to tell members of his staff that they had fallen short. After he started the job, his administrative assistant commented to him that whereas physicians leaving his predecessor's office often looked angry and disgruntled, now the same people leaving the same office were smiling. My colleague knew that he had that talent, but couldn't articulate how he did it. His colleagues (including me) could see that he would note the other's distress, acknowledge it, but not give in. If the other person intensified demands, he'd slow down, pause, reflect on what was really important, and then act. He had the presence of mind not to fall into the trap of escalation. His was a clear example of a healthy response to stress; he'd feel that he had done the right thing and he'd sleep well at night.

Not all of us have the natural skill that he did. Some of us need practice. Just as it's possible to practice mindfulness of your own mind, you can also practice mindfulness in relationships—interpersonal mindfulness. Earlier in the book I described how narratives—stories that doctors write about their difficult moments in practice—and deep listening can promote communication, reflection, and presence. Another dyadic contemplative practice is known as Insight Dialogue;[26] participants pair off and have a conversation, usually about a topic that has some personal salience, such as aging or illness or compassion or courage. But it's not an ordinary conversation. Participants are instructed to speak from the heart: first pause, open, and relax, then speak what comes first to mind, trusting that which comes spontaneously, to "listen deeply" and "speak the truth." The goal is to bring the clarity and mindfulness of silent meditation practice directly into conversations with others. Just as meditation helps focus the wandering mind through the practice of awareness of one's interior life, insight dialogues help participants be mindful of their own quality of listening and speaking.

Another interpersonal mindfulness technique is known as Appreciative Inquiry.[27] Here, an interviewer elicits from his or her partner a story of success amid adversity—a time when a positive attribute of the interviewee made a difference. By explicitly focusing on the positive, and having a partner help to maintain that focus, you can bring your strengths to new and unfamiliar situations. Originally conceived as a way of harnessing potential and cohesion in organizations, appreciative interviews start by promoting mindfulness in dialogue. Little is known about how these practices work on a psychological level, much less a neurobiological one. But we do know that people who are in dialogue tend to mirror each other's physiologies, movements, and even patterns of neural firing, likely mediated through mirror neurons. The frontiers of social neuroscience are now being stretched, and new research is exploring our capacity for shared mind, shared presence,[28] and intersubjectivity—and how these human capacities enable us to make deep and healing connections.

EIGHT LEAPS

In this final section of the chapter, I'll share my eight "leaps." Much like Zen koans, I carry these leaps with me in practice because they help me refocus, explore, grow, and begin again with each patient. I invite you, whether or not you're involved in health care, to find your own leaps: What is it that you face every day that is unresolved? What dilemmas and paradoxes do you face? Perhaps you'll see some parallels with your own work situation or your home life.

THE EIGHT LEAPS

From fragmented self to whole self
From othering to engagement
From objectivity to resonance
From detached concern to tenderness and steadiness
From self-protection to self-suspension
From well-being to resilience
From empathy to compassion
From whole mind to shared mind

The first leap I call **"from fragmented self to whole self."** I've become increasingly aware that I bring some positive parts of myself to my clinical work—I'm curious, analytic, and I try to be kind. Other parts of me—my artistic side, perhaps—tend to "reside" at my research office, at vacation spots, and at home. I take these divisions—rarely based on any conscious choice—for granted; sometimes they are appropriate, but sometimes they lead to a sense of fragmentation, of loss. I ask myself each day, "What parts of myself am I engaging in my care of this patient, right now?" And then: "Does it have to be that way?"

The second leap is **"from othering to engagement."** The physician-poet Jack Coulehan proposes two reasons why clinicians detach emotionally from patients—to maintain objectivity, and to avoid being overwhelmed by the patient's suffering.[29] To detach, I use a "doctorly" voice, construct the patient as an "other," "the person in the bed," someone "not like me." The patient inhabits the world of the sick; we, the world of the well. I've even caught myself assuming my doctorly voice with family members, effectively "othering" them, something that wins little affection. While to suggest that I can truly understand someone else's experience would be arrogant, I still can try to "learn from below," letting the patient guide me to an understanding of her experience. This is a process of shared imagination. The philosopher G. C. Spivak calls it a "no-holds-barred self-suspending leap into the other's sea—basically without preparation."[30] When I say, "I can only begin to imagine," to a patient who is seriously ill or distressed, the patient then becomes my teacher; I feel inquisitive and humble. This moral act opens me up to surprises and leads to new ways of understanding. I ask myself, "In what ways is this patient like me?"

The third leap is **"from objectivity to resonance."** In medical school I was trained to be an objective observer. I needed to discern whether a heart murmur is harsh-sounding enough to warrant an echocardiogram, whether a patient's story is coherent or contradictory, or whether I've done enough diagnostic testing for someone with a headache. Objectivity, though, is a stance that I never fully inhabited because it sometimes feels false. Clinical practice is always richer and more satisfying to me and my patients if there is some well-boundaried and heartfelt sharing of emotion.[31] I ask myself, "What would happen if I allowed greater emotional resonance, if I allowed myself to feel just a little bit more?" Here, no particular distance is the "correct" distance; rather, it is the asking of the question that is important.

A related leap is one **"from detached concern to tenderness and steadiness."** Tenderness is a quality of touch—both literal touch or feeling touched through communication. Steadiness is the mental stability to get one's work done—and done well. As Jack Coulehan notes, tenderness and steadiness support each other and don't have to be mutually exclusive.[32] I ask myself, "Can I be both tender and steady even if the seas are turbulent?"

The fifth leap, **"from self-protection to self-suspension,"** has to do with fear. One of my favorite children's books (and my kids' too) is *Doctor De Soto*, about a mouse who is a dentist.[33] His patient is a fox. This is clearly a dangerous relationship. While the fox is imagining eating the mouse, the mouse focuses on the painful tooth. The fox's desire to avoid pain trumps his impulse to eat the mouse. They are able to work together, despite their differences, at least until the pain stops. The mouse, though, doesn't want to take any chances and glues the fox's jaw (temporarily) shut just as he is finishing his work.

Children's books often contain great wisdom. Sometimes our fears as physicians are well justified. A patient of mine who had just completed parole for armed robbery and attempted murder gently requested that I falsify data about his HIV status so that he would be eligible for life insurance. He asked questions about my family; he seemed to know where I lived. I had reason to believe that he had access to a gun. I said no and frankly felt a bit afraid. Even when I'm faced with threats that are illusory, I adopt psychological distance and armor to protect myself.

A few months later I had to give terrible news to this same patient; his headaches and difficulty concentrating were due to progressive multifocal leukoencephalopathy, a rapidly fatal brain disease that is a complication of advanced AIDS. I was bracing for the pain of having to tell him the awfulness of it all; I didn't sleep well, dreaming that he'd hear the news and turn a gun on me, his family, or himself. Yet, the next day, he said that he knew that something was wrong; he was calm and grateful for my candor. I had become aware of how my self-preoccupation had overshadowed my ability to attend to him. I make a habit of asking myself, "Whom am I trying to protect?"

"From well-being to resilience"—the sixth leap—means that trying to achieve "work-life balance" might be misguided. Rather, by focusing on the task at hand I often find joy in the moment, curiosity amid despair, resilience when I feel I'm going to pieces. I let go of distinctions between work and nonwork and instead ask myself, "What do I need to do right now?" "What am I anticipating, looking forward to, prepared for?" "What if something else happens?"

The seventh leap, **"from empathy to compassion,"** is a reminder that even if I have an accurate understanding of a patient's suffering, it doesn't necessarily mean that I'm addressing it adequately. I make a practice of asking myself, "How can I choose to be compassionate in a way that makes a difference?"

The leaps so far have been about me, my mind, and the ways in which I can bring my whole mind to clinical care. The eighth leap takes me **"from whole mind to shared mind."** My clinical life is working with people—patients and their families, clinical teams, health care systems, communities. Shared mind is about being on the same wavelength, adopting a similar frame of reference even when we disagree. This doesn't always happen. I ask myself, "Is this me working alone or is this us working together?" and "Might greater sharing produce better care?"

12

Imagining a Mindful
Health Care System

A cord of three strands is not quickly broken.
—Ecclesiastes 4:12

Imagine that you went to bed tonight and woke tomorrow morning to find that the health care system was transformed. You have a health concern. Perhaps it's something serious or perhaps it's something minor. You call the office. You're amazed that you can contact your doctor and get an appointment the same day. When you arrive, the staff is attentive and courteous and knows you. You're astounded at the care you receive; it's technically proficient, and your clinicians are alert to your concerns. They're interested in who you are—your work, your home life, what's important to you. They help you make decisions, guided not only by the latest research but also by your values and clinical situation. You know that the various doctors, nurses, and other health professionals caring for you are talking to one another, anticipating your needs and making sure that the advice you get is consistent. Safety checks are in place so that you are confident that errors will be extraordinarily rare, and when they do occur, you get a full and complete explanation along with confidence that it won't happen again. Your care is efficient, affordable, and effective.

Imagine that although your doctor is busy, she listens carefully to your concerns. She doesn't interrupt. You feel cared for as a person, not merely as a case or a problem to be solved. She seeks your opinions and encourages you to ask questions and express concerns. She doesn't hide behind her expertise and makes you feel that no question is too simple. She talks with you, not at you. Your health care team provides information and support so that you can participate in decisions regarding your care to the degree that you wish. You have a voice in the aspects of health care that matter most and your time isn't wasted with bureaucratic and administrative hassles. You feel that your health care team provides not only technical expertise but also emotional support when you need it.

Imagine that your doctor feels a sense of meaning in her work. Her work is difficult, stressful, and demanding, but your doctor has the self-awareness, mindfulness, and resilience to stay on top of things. Her meaningful relationships with patients sustain her through the workweek. She has enough control over scheduling and the organization of the office that she feels that she can do a good job. When dealing with the most difficult moments—when losing a patient, when witnessing needless suffering, when considering what might have contributed to a serious error, when making difficult ethical choices—she feels resilient and supported.

This utopian vision of health care is shared by some of those who have the greatest influence in health care today. Don Berwick, M.D., formerly head of Medicare and Medicaid during the Obama administration, coined the "triple aim" of health care—better health care experiences for patients, better health outcomes for the population, and lower cost. Since then, family physicians Tom Bodenheimer and Christine Sinsky have added a fourth aim: improving the work lives of clinicians and staff who provide care. These aims have been embraced, at least in name, by an increasing number of health care organizations nationally.[1]

I am a physician and not an organizational consultant, a CEO, or a manager. I take care of patients, one at a time. It took me a long time to realize that health care organizations have as much influence on my patients' health as I do. Now, with current changes in health care, that reality has become apparent to anyone who has contact with the health care system. But health care organizations aren't all the same. Only some truly embrace a vision of health care in which patients receive care that is effective, efficient, and affordable while sustaining the viability of the health care workforce and make real efforts to achieve those aims.[2] Too often, though, health care institutions think only about productivity and throughput and don't take into account what helps clinicians and staff to be at their best.

Just like people, organizations themselves can be described as attentive, curious, responsive, and present—or not. They have the equivalent of top-down attention based on the goals of the organization as well as bottom-up attention, triggered by unexpected opportunities and challenges. And just like individuals, organizations pay selective attention to some things and ignore others, base decisions on incomplete knowledge, aren't completely rational in their decision making, and muddle through when decisions are complex. Organizations have habits of mind, the collective habits that constitute an organization's culture. Organizations can be described as mindful or less than mindful. In the transformation that I envision, health care organizations would promote mindfulness of individuals, health care teams, and of the organizational culture itself—down to how meetings are conducted, how information is communicated, and what values and behaviors are highlighted. They would create the conditions within which mindfulness could grow. The challenge is how to make this all happen.

COLLECTIVE MIND

The idea of mindfulness in organizations is not new. Karl Weick, at the University of Michigan's Ross School of Business, first described the qualities of so-called high-reliability organizations in the 1990s. He visited aircraft carriers, nuclear power plants, airplane cockpits, and other settings in which a small error spells catastrophe. In the beginning of one of his articles, he asks the reader to imagine life on the flight deck of an aircraft carrier.[3] Planes take off and land on a slippery flight deck at half the intervals that would be allowed at a civilian airport. This is all happening on a ship that is rocking from side to side with its radar turned off to avoid detection—and the whole operation is run by a group of twenty-year-olds. One glitch and the pilot, the airplane, and the ship go up in flames. Yet, errors are rare. It does not take much imagination to see the parallels between flight decks and busy urban trauma centers and operating rooms. However, in medicine we do far worse, with over one hundred thousand deaths per year due to medical error, and not nearly enough improvement in the fifteen years since the publication of a highly publicized report, *To Err Is Human*, by the Institute of Medicine.[4]

Over the next twenty-five years, Weick and his colleagues identified features of what he called "high-reliability organizations" and was curious about how these organizations do their work—what they do, how they think and solve problems, and how they create organizational culture. Mindfulness was the missing link. Along with his colleague Kathleen Sutcliffe, Weick examined how organizations—as if the organizations were organisms—stand to gain by becoming more attentive, responsive, and reliable, and by learning to balance routine with innovation. They showed how freeing the mind from the concepts that constrain our thinking, the importance of beginner's mind, and the concept of emptiness were as fundamental to well-functioning organizations as they were for well-functioning individuals.[5] Weick advanced five basic principles of what he called "collective mind," "organizational mindfulness," and "organizational attention."[6]

First, Weick asserts, you need to be *preoccupied with failure*. There are just too many ways that things can go wrong, each unique and often unpredictable. That's why it's important, in Weick and Sutcliffe's words, to learn how to manage the unexpected—being prepared to be unprepared. This preparation should be part of institutional culture.[7]

Weick and Sutcliffe's second principle is to *be reluctant to simplify*. Just as individuals get derailed by using mental shortcuts, teams and organizations do too. When Mr. Laszlo, the patient I discussed in chapter 2, came in with a painful shoulder, three out of three clinicians sought a simple answer that was logical—and wrong. When my friend Gary went to the emergency room with urinary obstruction (chapter 4), the nurses and doctors caring for him made the same kind of mistake. They picked the most convenient explanation. They didn't question it; their minds were too crowded and there was too much pressure to move on to the next patient. In the ER, there might even have been an underlying organizational culture, one in which having a quick answer—any answer—was rewarded and deeper cognitive processing was not. Those caring for Gary lacked attention and presence, not just individually, but collectively.

Weick and Sutcliffe's third principle is *sensitivity to operations*—management speak for what in medicine is called situation awareness. Here, health care institutions have made progress. In most institutions, clinical teams who work in hospitals—such as in the OR, the ICU, and the labor and delivery floor—undergo team training to help members speak up when they observe a problem. Even when people are not part of a team, they're encouraged to speak up. The person who mops the floors might have better insight into why infections are rampant in an ICU than the director of infection control. Weick suggests that safety be given higher priority than efficiency—not just in word, but in deed. This involves a mindful redirection of attention toward things that might otherwise be ignored.

Commitment to resilience, Weick and Sutcliffe's fourth principle, is more than bouncing back. Like individual resilience, organizational resilience depends on learning and growing from crises, and working outside people's comfort zones. You need teams of *adaptive* experts, people who can learn from the past but also know when to let go of it.

Their last recommendation is the one that surprised me the most, in a pleasant way. Weick and Sutcliffe call for *greater anarchy in organizations*. In healthy organizations, they claim, decisions should be made by the most appropriate member of the hierarchy and shouldn't have to be delayed until they come to the attention of the leadership. Weick and Sutcliffe are not talking about total anarchy here, but about loosening the boundaries just a bit so that more decisions are made by the people closest to the problem. These make routines and structures in the organization a bit more fluid.[8] In my office, medical assistants take patients' pulse, temperature, and blood pressure and ask them what's bothering them when they arrive. The most helpful medical assistants are the ones who note that something is different—the patient's blood pressure is lower or higher than it should be—and interrupt me to bring it to my attention immediately rather than just recording it in the chart. At the other extreme was a medical assistant who recorded the patient's chief concern as "chest pain," entered it into the medical record correctly, then left the patient to wait in a room for a half hour until his physician saw him. The patient was having a heart attack. The medical assistant's failure was not merely an individual's lapse or irresponsibility; it reflected poor training and a culture that didn't reinforce mindfulness.[9]

QUALITY AND SAFETY

Promoting quality in health care should build on a foundation of individual mindfulness and at the same time develop organizational mindfulness. Institutions should be structured so that collective vigilance is the norm, so that it matters less if any one individual suffers a lapse in attention. For example, one difficult problem in health care has been preventing falls among the elderly. Falls are common, and if the patient is injured or in pain, she ends up immobilized. Even after a few days in bed, elderly patients lose strength and require additional rehabilitation, and even still they might not ever get back on their feet. Immobilization leads to infections and blood clots, and mortality can be as high as 50 percent in the ensuing year. Preventing falls takes collective vigilance. Nurses need to be alert to when patients are unstable or are trying to get out of bed when they shouldn't. When a bed alarm goes off, the response has to be quick and coordinated, as it often takes more than one person to get the patient to safety. One factor in reducing falls, according to Timothy Vogus at Vanderbilt University, is collective mindfulness.

He studied ninety-five nursing units to see if scores on a mindfulness survey, assessing the five components defined by Weick and Sutcliffe, would predict on which nursing units patients fell. Those units whose members *collectively* scored higher had fewer falls—and, also of note, fewer medication errors.[10]

Health care organizations should consider the human capacity for attention when designing clinical work spaces, ones free of frequent interruptions and distractions. When I'm working in the emergency room, where the decibel level is high and there's a potential distraction every few seconds, I mentally block out ambient sounds so that I can pay attention to my patient. It's exhausting. When it comes time to write my notes on the computer, I'm faced with a choice—wall myself off with varying degrees of success or go to a quieter space on another unit, a five-minute walk and five flights of stairs away. There has to be a better way. Mindful workspace design can make paying attention possible.

HUMAN CONVERSATIONS

Health care institutions can create the conditions for caring and compassion. Health care consultant and internist Tony Suchman says that part of the answer is in moving from a command-and-control leadership style to one that is more relationship centered.[11] Suchman describes relationship-centered leadership as a style that honors the unique individual contributions of each member while helping them contribute to the overall mission. Mindful leaders enshrine the human side of medicine in hospital culture, provide space for meaningful conversations among members of the organization, and discover employees' untapped strengths. Suchman takes a radical view of organizations—that they are no more than a collection of conversations among people, setting the stage for appreciative inquiry and other methods to enhance motivation and self-awareness, promote effective teamwork, and help individuals sustain a sense of vision, purpose, and meaning.[12]

Leaders should promote inquiry, awareness, and attention to

things that matter and that the organization values. Over the past two years, I spent several days at a large Catholic health care system and was the keynote speaker at a conference of the Catholic Health Association. I was struck with several cultural differences between Catholic health systems and the secular world of university hospitals. First, they had an explicit commitment to caring and compassion. In chapter 7, I described how I checked out hospital mission statements looking for mention of suffering; at the same time I also looked for the word *compassion*. Nearly all of the Catholic health systems mentioned compassion explicitly, whereas almost none of the secular hospital systems did. Perhaps where the word *compassion* is spoken more often, it is enacted more often. But these are interesting times. Catholic hospitals in the United States have traditionally cared for everyone, even those with no means to pay. Historically they were run by nuns. Now they are typically run by lay leadership and are experiencing growing pains as they compete for market share and merge with other hospitals. However, I was intrigued by a role that they still had in their administrative structure and that I had not seen in other hospitals—directors of "formation." These people orient health care workers to consider such questions as "Where do I find meaning each day?" "What grounds this work?" "To what are we called together?" and "How must we respond?" I find these questions important, regardless of one's spiritual orientation. They address the technical as well as the existential, ethical, and social aspects of care. These hospitals' commitment to formation and mission is right on the mark. I found it particularly refreshing after having visited with institutions whose investment in compassion is little more than a sticker on a white lab coat that says I CARE.[13]

Ken Schwartz was a successful Boston attorney who represented health care institutions. He was diagnosed with metastatic cancer at age forty and died ten months later, but not before recognizing what was most important—and sometimes most lacking—in the health care he received. He published his account in the *Boston Globe* and pointed to the small acts of kindness that made "the unbearable bearable." His final wish was to create an organization that would nurture compassion, caregiver-patient relationships, and humane care. Founded in 1995, shortly before Ken Schwartz's death, the Schwartz Center for Compassionate Healthcare[14] has a signature program called Schwartz Rounds, which is currently in place at over five hundred health care institutions in North America and the UK. Schwartz Rounds focus on a patient with complex medical issues that require an interdisciplinary approach. Each session assembles a patient's care team, which may include physicians, nurses, therapists, chaplains, and others who have meaningful contact with the patient and his family. Panelists talk openly about the difficulties they've encountered caring for the patient. Sometimes the patient or a family member is present to add to the discussion.

In a recent Schwartz Rounds at my hospital, a mother reflected on her experiences during a recent hospitalization for her severely disabled son, one of many hospitalizations for seizures, pneumonia, and weight loss. The care team, including a pediatric geneticist, the ICU physician, a nurse, a social worker, and a chaplain, described the child's predicament, how they each were affected by his suffering, knowing that little could be done to reverse his decline. Importantly, the 150 attendees, from a wide variety of disciplines and specialties, as well as the patient's mother, discussed how the health care system could best support the family. Discussions like this, in a well-attended forum, rarely happened in hospitals until the Schwartz Center started supporting them. Now, in our institution and others, Schwartz Rounds occur monthly and are a source of community building for the medical and nursing staff. A few years ago, Beth Lown, an internist and medical director at the Schwartz Center, assessed the impact of Schwartz Rounds.[15] Those who had attended reported deeper insight into the emotional lives of patients and caregivers. They communicated better—verbally and nonverbally—and felt more equipped to respond to patients' needs with compassion. They were more energized about their work. They felt less stressed and isolated and more open to providing and accepting support. They became more mindful by learning to speak from the heart, just as the panelists had done.

The Arnold P. Gold Foundation has a similar mission, and has pioneered the "white coat ceremony," conducted at nearly all of the medical schools in North America, to mark the transition from student to healer. By asking students to develop and commit to a set of professional vows, the ceremony brings students' awareness, at the beginning of their careers, squarely to the values, attitudes, and attributes that they each bring to the profession—a guidepost for more mindful, humane care.

A CORD OF THREE STRANDS

It seems so sensible that quality of care, quality of caring, and clinician resilience would be synergistic. Even in these difficult times in health care, I see more and more health professionals tending to the soil in which their focused attention, curiosity, creativity, compassion, and resilience can grow. Yet, they are doing this in spite of their organizations, which they continue to find unsympathetic and unsupportive. Creating mindful organizations starts with respecting the clinicians who work there. Organizations should provide opportunities during the workday for clinicians to grow professionally and not make those offerings add-ons to an already overcrowded day. At some institutions, self-awareness and mindfulness constitute an essential part of the required curriculum for students and residents,[16] and these institutions frame self-awareness as essential to good patient care. Each of us has a lot at stake. When I teach medical students, I do so knowing that they represent the future of medicine. I assume that each student will become the doctor that I might encounter in the emergency room if I have another kidney stone, in the oncology clinic if I have cancer, or in the hospital if I need surgery. In fact, this has happened; some of my students have been my doctors. And I am hopeful. While some medical school graduates consider medicine as nothing more than a job, when I informally polled several medical school classes recently, the majority had done some kind of contemplative practice and see value in it for themselves as professionals. They see medicine as deeply meaningful work.

Attending—where you focus your precious attentional resources—is a choice, a moral choice. When I started thinking about mindful practice in medicine twenty years ago, I saw it as an individual commitment to be more attentive and curious, have a beginner's mind, and be present. I described the skills necessary to move from being a mere expert to a master, with the associated insight, perspective, and creativity. Now I see the project as much larger. Like the African proverb about raising a child, mindful practice takes a village. Having a community of colleagues, peers, and others who share a vision of mindful practice makes it possible. In clinical care the beneficiaries are our patients, who themselves may bring attention and awareness to their own work, whether they are artists, schoolteachers, bus drivers, or lawyers. Mindfulness is an aspiration of an increasing number of individuals and large educational and corporate institutions that comprise our society. I believe that now it is possible, with the right resolve, to have health care infused with and guided by mindful practice. A cord of three strands—individual, collective, and institutional—is not quickly broken.

Acknowledgments

Attending could never have been realized without the efforts of a few key people. Most notable is Rebecca Gradinger, who through her confidence in me led me to find my voice and sustain the passion and energy for the book. She is an agent extraordinaire, passionate advocate, and tough critic, who never stopped believing in this book even when I was mired in doubt. She answered e-mails at noon and midnight and kept me focused on who I am and what I could give. She and her team at Fletcher & Company, including Jennifer Herrera and Veronica Goldstein, were incredibly supportive. Rebecca introduced me to my editor, Shannon Welch, whose passion for the topic, thoughtful editorial guidance, and commitment helped to make *Attending* the best it could be. Along with her remarkable team at Scribner, including her associate editor, John Glynn, and editor-in-chief, Colin Harrison, she shaped the manuscript so that it spoke with greater clarity and coherence. For their efforts and commitment I'll be forever grateful.

I want to thank Gail Gazelle, Tula Karras, and Paula Derrow, who coached me early on, as I was just conceiving the book. My friend and medical school classmate Dan Siegel and my palliative care colleague Ira Byock gave me important advice about the publishing world, and my friend and college classmate Ron Siegel gave me the real skinny on books and editors and agents. He read, and hated, my first draft of a proposal, advising me that readers want the richness of stories, not merely sterile ideas. As I was drafting the book proposal, Arthur Frank, Jon Kabat-Zinn, Tim Quill, and

Marc Lesser also offered support, enthusiasm, and helpful critiques through the eyes of those who'd been through it all before. Steven Henry Boldt, Mahala Ruppel, Esther Brown, Maria Milella, Betsy Frarey, and Deborah Fox all read the manuscript in its entirety and provided invaluable editorial suggestions for style, grammar, and sense. Thanks to you all.

I was amazed and grateful when friends and colleagues came out of the woodwork offering to read the manuscript in its entirety and provide specific critiques and impressions, most notably Andy Elliot and Bill Ventres, accomplished writers and busy people. Andy brought a reader's eye to each sentence and reminded me that I was writing to reach out to others as well as to understand myself. Bill provided inspiration, thoughtful critiques, and gentle prods to "get real" when my thinking became too abstract and academic. Saskia Hendriks, a fellow researcher at the Brocher Foundation, provided insightful comments that led to important changes in the first two chapters of the manuscript.

I am a physician and not a neuroscientist, and although I had read hundreds of articles about the neurobiology of attention, resilience, attachment, compassion, and curiosity, I needed help reconciling competing ways of understanding how the brain and the mind work. Al Kaszniak and Jud Brewer read the portions of the manuscript about neuroscience research, correcting my misconceptions and getting me as up-to-date as one can be in a field that is evolving rapidly. Olga Klimecki was kind enough to explain the procedures and limitations of functional-imaging research, including her research on empathy, compassion, and conflict. Conversations with Amishi Jha helped me to understand more deeply the mechanisms of attention, Eric Nestler and Stephen Southwick helped interpret research on resilience, and Jean Decety and Beth Lown helped me to understand better the neurobiology and psychology of empathy and compassion. Anthropologist and Zen teacher Roshi Joan Halifax introduced me to the work of Carl Batson and Nancy Eisenberg, whose theories of empathy, sympathy, and compassion deeply influenced my thinking. Evan Thompson, a philosopher of mind and cognitive scientist, expanded my notion of what minds could do and be, and my Rochester colleague Paul Duberstein introduced me to the idea of collaborative cognition, which informed my ideas about shared mind. Chris Lyddy and Darren Good helped me to develop ideas about organizational mindfulness and sent me literature from the world of business and organizational management that might be applied to medicine. Yishai Mintzker brought to my attention the shared etymologies of *meditation* and *medicine*.

Several chapters represent a shared inspiration. I owe a debt of gratitude to Larry Dyche, who badgered me for months to respond to his offer to cowrite an article on curiosity just as I was beginning to think about writing this book, and the article we wrote together in 2011 influenced chapter 3. Similarly, Tony Back's imprint on chapter 7 and my understanding of suffering is profound, as represented in a 2015 article we coauthored. Jordan Silberman and Dan Siegel helped me develop ideas about self-monitoring, which influenced much of how I frame mindfulness for clinical audiences. The focus on difficult decisions (chapter 6), suffering (chapter 7), compassion (chapter 8), errors and grief (chapter 9), and burnout and resilience (chapter 10) closely parallels the curriculum that Mick Krasner and I developed collaboratively for educational programs for students, residents, and practicing clinicians. I am grateful to all these colleagues for their generosity in sharing their ideas and letting me bring them from the academic realm to the public eye.

I am grateful for the gift of time. My department chair in the Department of Family Medicine at the University of Rochester, Tom Campbell, and Vice-Chair Susan McDaniel, advocated for my 2014 sabbatical—supported by the University of Rochester— during which I monkishly developed the book proposal. I am also grateful for the gift of space. The Brocher Foundation, just outside Geneva, Switzerland, is devoted to the social aspects of medicine, and enthusiastically supported my writing by providing a room and a tranquil study overlooking Lac Léman to complete the first draft of this book in February 2016. Several foundations supported the background work for the book through their funding of my time to develop, implement, and evaluate the educational programs that demonstrated effectiveness of mindful practice training on clinician well-being, resilience, and quality of care they could provide. I am particularly grateful to the Arthur Vining Davis Foundations, the Arnold P. Gold Foundation, the Maria Tussi Kluge and John W. Kluge Foundation, the Mannix Fund, and the Physicians Foundation for Health Systems Excellence.

Several teachers have had an enduring influence. My fifth-grade teacher, Marguerite Britton, ran her classroom as a democratic organization focused on identifying individuals' learning needs and taught me about presence amid chaos, much to my enrichment and the school principal's dismay. In college, my main influences were Randy Huntsberry, who introduced me to emptiness and mindfulness, and how mindfulness and stillness can happen in movement; Ken Maue, music and philosophical visionary; and the late Jon Barlow, who could make connections among anything, including baseball, Charles Ives, and John Ford, and between sixteenth-century English keyboard music and southern-Indian mridangam drumming. They all taught me that the way you see the world is limited only by your expectations and imagination. In medical school, my inspirations were psychiatrists Peter Reich and Les Havens, both humanists bucking the tides of psychoanalytic rigidity and biological reductionism, and later, in Rochester, George Engel, who taught me how to observe and ask. I wish they were still of this world so that I could thank them.

After I finished my medical training, my colleagues became my teachers. The late Ian McWhinney, family physician and philosopher, lived and breathed patient-centered care. My Catalan colleague Francesc Borrell-Carrió has been one of my most treasured intellectual partners and critics. He introduced me to pragmatist philosophers in my own backyard—John Dewey and William James—and has a way of gently questioning and challenging me to be as clear as I can be. David Leach, another Aristotelian, showed me the logic behind breaking rules in the name of wisdom, an idea dear to my anarchist heart, and how organizations themselves could become more mindful in the process. Conversations with Stuart and Hubert Dreyfus, Kevin Eva, Brian Hodges, and Carol-Anne Moulton strongly shaped my concept of expertise in medicine and how to know when you have it. While he was the senior associate dean for medical education at the University of Rochester, Ed Hundert provided the opportunities for me to lay the intellectual groundwork about how we understand and assess competence. Lucy Candib helped me understand the meaning of suffering and oppression and what doctors can do about them. From Susan McDaniel, Dave Seaburn, and Pieter LeRoux I learned a family-systems orientation and family-of-origin awareness that suffuses every moment of my practice, teaching me that there is never just one patient in the room. Peter Franks taught me to adopt healthy skepticism about my own senses and convictions, especially those I hold most strongly. My greatest teachers have often been my patients, who, for confidentiality, must remain unnamed, yet I am grateful for their generosity, tolerance, and patience with me when I was off the mark.

The mindful practice programs that I describe in this book were the collective brainchild of my colleague Mick Krasner and me, with considerable input from Fred Marshall, Tim Quill, Scott McDonald, Stephen Liben, Patricia Lück, Shauna Shapiro, Tony Back, and Heidi Schwarz. Mick, the intuitive, spontaneous extrovert, offers the perfect complement to my analytical, conceptual way of seeing the world, and our educational programming is truly an example of shared mind. I am grateful for intellectual leadership, inspiration, and guidance from Jon Kabat-Zinn and Saki Santorelli and their colleagues at the Center for Mindfulness in Medicine, Health Care, and Society at the University of Massachusetts; from Rita Charon and Tom Inui, who helped me develop the narrative medicine components of the mindful practice programs; and from Penny Williamson, who shared her wisdom about appreciative inquiry. I thank Michael Zimler, Ed Brown, Reb Anderson, Richard Baker, Joseph Goldstein, and Christopher Titmuss for their generosity in helping me develop a meditation practice. I have been deeply influenced by many other conversations with teachers, mentors, friends, and colleagues over the past forty years, and to name them all would be impossible. Sometimes I may have forgotten the source of an idea, but that makes me no less grateful.

Acknowledgments

By far my deepest thanks go to my wife, Deborah. Her clarity about what is important, her insistence that I speak from the heart — my heart and no one else's — her frank critiques, her bullshit detector, her ability to size up people, her willingness to drop everything to help me think of just the right word, and her ability to channel me even when we are continents apart are extraordinary. She is my best editor and most loving critic. She tolerated my grouchiness, brought me tea and ripe pears, and even took over cooking dinner, normally my task, so I could write uninterrupted. My children, Eli and Malka, have helped me see the world through new eyes, and I am moved to tears by their emulation of those parts of me that give me joy, and by their tolerance of those parts that I'm not always proud of. And my parents, Joan and the late Jules Epstein, were totally mystified when my first-semester college transcript listed a course called Emptiness, but kept paying the tuition, trusting that I was doing something valuable even if they couldn't understand it, and didn't flinch when I announced I'd be a harpsichordist, then a Zen student, then a musicologist, then a chef, then an acupuncturist, and then a doctor. Their confidence in me was unwavering, and they knew it would all work out somehow.

Appendix: Attention Practice

In the beginning, meditation—like any new habit—takes practice. First, the effort is in just doing it—making time and being consistent. Frequently, the next challenge is stabilizing one's attention, learning how to be in the present moment and how not to drift into mind-wandering or rumination. After sustained practice, meditation becomes effortless. The hard-won focus and awareness feel natural and simple. For me (and although I've practiced for decades, I make no claim to being an advanced practitioner), meditation is a habit, like brushing my teeth, so much so that the day would feel incomplete without it.

The instructions for both focused attention practice and open awareness practice start with posture; it should be comfortable and "dignified." If sitting in a chair, you should be upright with feet on the floor; if on a cushion, you can be cross-legged or kneeling. Training need not be done sitting; practices can be done while walking, standing, or even lying down (a bit trickier because of the tendency to fall asleep!).

In Zen training, focused attention practice comes first, whereas in Vipassana training (otherwise called mindfulness meditation), both focused attention and open awareness are introduced early on. Focused attention starts with an awareness of the breath. In the Zen tradition, trainees are taught to count breaths—one, two, three, and up to ten, restarting at one and continuing to ten, then back to one, and so forth. In the Vipassana tradition, the focus is on awareness of the breath, and counting is not emphasized; instead attention is directed toward watching its rhythm, depth, and speed. You don't try to control the breath in any way, but rather just notice how it is deep or shallow, fast or slow, regular or irregular.

For open awareness practice, the instructions are a bit different. You don't necessarily focus on the breath, a mantra, or anything else. Rather, you assume an open, receptive, nonjudgmental awareness of all physical sensations, thoughts, and feelings that may be transpiring—whether they arise from within the body or from the external world—without any attempt to alter them in any way. It's like watching a movie and being the main character at the same time—it's observing the observer observing the observed.[1] Open awareness involves naming those sensations: "Oh, I'm feeling my foot itch" or "Oh, there was just a loud noise." Similarly, one can name emotions as they arise: "I'm noticing that I'm feeling angry"—or sad or frustrated. Naming emotions helps us engage in first-person inquiry, be curious, and respond to emotions intelligently, even if our first reactions are avoidance or annoyance.

If you're starting on your own, choose one practice and stick with it. Get any of the dozens of audio-recordings, apps, or books, or go to a workshop.[2] Your choice of practice may depend on whether you can find a partner or a group with whom you can practice—just as with exercise or any other lifestyle change. You may want to dive right in with twenty to forty minutes a day or start more slowly and increase as you can; even five minutes in the morning can make a difference. Importantly, be gentle with yourself—if you're counting breaths and you can never get beyond three or find yourself at 142, gently bring yourself back to the task. A kind smile always helps.

You may remember two other practices mentioned earlier in the book—the body scan (chapter 3) and metta meditation (chapter 8). For these practices a guide can be helpful—either in person, or via one of the innumerable guided meditations available on the Web.

Notes

1. BEING MINDFUL

1 Even if one kidney had sustained permanent damage, given Jake's young age, the other kidney would be highly likely to assume greater functioning over time and his kidney function would normalize—just as it does in people who donate a kidney for transplantation.

2 For descriptions of cognitive traps, see articles by emergency-room physician and decision scientist Patrick Croskerry: P. Croskerry, "The Importance of Cognitive Errors in Diagnosis and Strategies to Minimize Them," *Academic Medicine* 78(8) (2003): 775–80; P. Croskerry and G. Norman, "Overconfidence in Clinical Decision Making," *American Journal of Medicine* 121(5) (2008): S24–S29; P. Croskerry, "A Universal Model of Diagnostic Reasoning," *Academic Medicine* 84(8) (2009): 1022–28; P. Croskerry, "Context Is Everything or How Could I Have Been That Stupid?," *Healthcare Quarterly* 12 (2009): e171–e176; P. Croskerry, "From Mindless to Mindful Practice—Cognitive Bias and Clinical Decision Making," *New England Journal of Medicine* 368(26) (2013): 2445–48; and descriptions of Croskerry's practice in J. E. Groopman, *How Doctors Think* (New York: Houghton Mifflin, 2007).

3 For a detailed discussion of the holistic and multifaceted nature of professional competence of clinicians, see R. M. Epstein and E. M. Hundert, "Defining and Assessing Professional Competence," *JAMA* 287(2) (2002): 226–35; and R. M. Epstein, "Mindful Practice," *JAMA* 282(9) (1999): 833–39.

4 Philosopher Michael Polanyi calls this subsidiary awareness, that which is just beneath the surface, accessible to consciousness, but which is kept tacit so that we do not stumble. A pianist, for example, if asked to constantly be aware of each finger movement, would stumble more than if those movements were maintained outside awareness. See M. Polanyi, *Personal Knowledge: Towards a Post-critical Philosophy* (Chicago: University of Chicago Press, 1974); and M. Polanyi, *The Tacit Dimension* (Gloucester, MA: Peter Smith, 1983). A related construct is pre-attentive processing, in which the brain "selects" which of many sources to attend to. See J. H. Austin, *Zen and the Brain: Toward an Understanding of Meditation and Consciousness* (Cambridge, MA: MIT Press, 1998). Another related construct is process knowledge, knowing

how to do things, often tacit when it involves learned behaviors such as tying knots for a surgeon, riding a bicycle, playing scales for a pianist, etc., a useful construct in education. See M. Eraut, *Developing Professional Knowledge and Competence* (London: Falmer Press, 1994).

5 C.-A. Moulton and R. M. Epstein, "Self-Monitoring in Surgical Practice: Slowing Down When You Should," in *Surgical Education: Theorising an Emerging Domain*, ed. H. Fry and R. Kneebone (New York: Springer, 2011), chap. 10, 169–82; and C.-A. Moulton et al., "Slowing Down When You Should: A New Model of Expert Judgment," *Academic Medicine RIME: Proceedings of the Forty-Sixth Annual Conference* 82(10) (2007): S109–S116.

6 In all fairness, I don't know whether Mehta was curious or not. Perhaps he was, in which case it was an internal experience that he didn't share. Reich's curiosity was visible.

7 I am grateful to Randy Huntsberry, PhD, the professor for this course and others I took while at Wesleyan University. He had a strongly positive transformative effect on me and others.

8 J. Kabat-Zinn, *Wherever You Go, There You Are: Mindfulness Meditation in Everyday Life* (New York: Hyperion, 1994).

9 More accurately, Nagarjuna, the second-century Buddhist philosopher, would propose a fourfold paradox—to see yourself as fallible, to see yourself as infallible, to see yourself as both fallible and infallible, and finally to see yourself as neither fallible nor infallible. See F. J. Streng, *Emptiness: A Study in Religious Meaning* (Nashville, TN: Abingdon Press, 1967).

10 G. L. Engel, "The Need for a New Medical Model: A Challenge for Biomedicine," *Science* 196(4286) (1977): 129–36.

11 G. L. Engel, "The Clinical Application of the Biopsychosocial Model," *American Journal of Psychiatry* 137(5) (1980): 535–44; and G. L. Engel, "From Biomedical to Biopsychosocial: Being Scientific in the Human Domain," *Psychosomatics* 38(6) (1997): 521–28.

12 In the 1950s, British psychiatrist Michael Balint pioneered a group format in which general practitioners would discuss difficult cases. Through deep inquiry, Balint would help the GPs uncover otherwise hidden emotional reactions to patients that could affect the care they provided their patients—positively and negatively. He firmly believed that the person of the physician was as important a therapeutic agent as the drugs physicians could prescribe. See M. Balint, *The Doctor, His Patient, and the Illness* (New York: International Universities Press, 1957); I. R. McWhinney, "Fifty Years On: The Legacy of Michael Balint," *British Journal of General Practice* 49 (1999): 418–19; and L. Scheingold, "Balint Work in England: Lessons for American Family Medicine," *Journal of Family Practice* 26(3) (1988): 315–20.

13 Family-of-origin groups explore the influences of one's own family—history, values, beliefs, use of language, degree of cohesion, etc.—on one's clinical work. See S. H. McDaniel, T. L. Campbell, and D. B. Seaburn, *Family-Oriented Primary Care: A Manual for Medical Providers* (New York: Springer-Verlag, 1990); R. M. Epstein, "Physician Know Thy Family: Looking at One's Family of Origin as a Method of Physician Self-Awareness," *Medical Encounter* 8(1) (1991): 9; S. H. McDaniel and J. Landau-Stanton, "Family-of-Origin Work

and Family Therapy Skills Training: Both-And," *Family Process* 30(4) (1991): 459–71; and M. Mengel, "Physician Ineffectiveness due to Family-of-Origin Issues," *Family Systems Medicine* 5(2) (1987): 176–90.

14 Personal-awareness groups, developed by the American Academy on Communication in Health Care, are a group format for physicians to explore their inner lives and relationships, based on the work of psychologist Carl Rogers. D. H. Novack et al., "Calibrating the Physician: Personal Awareness and Effective Patient Care," *JAMA* 278(6) (1997): 502–9; T. E. Quill and P. R. Williamson, "Healthy Approaches to Physician Stress," *Archives of Internal Medicine* 150(9) (1990): 1857–61; and R. C. Smith et al., "Efficacy of a One-Month Training Block in Psychosocial Medicine for Residents: A Controlled Study," *Journal of General Internal Medicine* 6(6) (1991): 535–43.

15 I am grateful to David Sperber, who led a personal-awareness group for family medicine residents for thirty years, and to David Seaburn, Susan McDaniel, Pieter LeRoux, and others, who led family-of-origin reflection groups during my fellowship training.

16 Concepts that I explored included personal knowledge, procedural knowledge, process knowledge, tacit knowledge, self-reflection, reflective practitioner, reflection-on-action, reflection-in-action, knowledge-in-action, intersubjectivity, enaction, and more, all cited in Epstein, "Mindful Practice."

17 Publications in the late 1990s began to focus on the interior lives of physicians and the impact of self-awareness on clinical practice. See S. L. Shapiro, G. E. Schwartz, and G. Bonner, "Effects of Mindfulness-Based Stress Reduction on Medical and Premedical Students," *Journal of Behavioral Medicine* 21(6) (1998): 581–99; S. L. Shapiro and G. E. Schwartz, "Mindfulness in Medical Education: Fostering the Health of Physicians and Medical Practice," *Integrative Medicine* 1(3) (1998): 93–94; R. C. Smith et al., "Teaching Self-Awareness Enhances Learning about Patient-Centered Interviewing," *Academic Medicine* 74(11) (1999): 1242–48; D. H. Novack, R. M. Epstein, and R. H. Paulsen, "Toward Creating Physician-Healers: Fostering Medical Students' Self-Awareness, Personal Growth, and Well-Being," *Academic Medicine* 74(5) (1999): 516–20; D. H. Novack et al., "Personal Awareness and Professional Growth: A Proposed Curriculum," *Medical Encounter* 13(3) (1997): 2–7; and Novack et al., "Calibrating the Physician."

18 Epstein and Hundert, "Defining and Assessing Professional Competence."

19 The Comprehensive Assessment program for medical students emphasizes the skills of diagnosis and treatment but also the capacity of students to reflect and be self-aware. Students continue to say that it is one of most formative parts of their medical school career, and it gives me hope that students are hungry to know themselves more deeply. See R. M. Epstein et al., "Comprehensive Assessment of Professional Competence: The Rochester Experiment," *Teaching and Learning in Medicine* 16(2) (2004): 186–96.

20 Epstein, "Mindful Practice."

21 M. C. Beach et al., "A Multicenter Study of Physician Mindfulness and Health Care Quality," *Annals of Family Medicine* 11(5) (2013): 421–28. Beach assessed physicians' (lack of) mindfulness using a standard mindfulness survey that included items such as "I tend to walk quickly to where I am going with-

out paying attention to what I experience along the way" or "I find myself listening to someone with one ear, doing something else at the same time" or "I frequently forget a person's name shortly after we meet." Although it is odd to think that one could self-rate one's own mindfulness, the surveys do predict what most would consider to be mindful behaviors and correlate with more experience with meditation. P. Grossman, "On Measuring Mindfulness in Psychosomatic and Psychological Research," *Journal of Psychosomatic Research* 64(4) (2008): 405–8.

22 I discovered a like-minded colleague in Rochester, Dr. Mick Krasner, and the two of us spearheaded workshops and seminars in mindful practice for physicians, residents, students, and medical educators in Rochester. These have blossomed into programs on six continents. Several foundations funded us to help make those ideas a reality. The 1999 *JAMA* "Mindful Practice" article has been cited in the medical literature over a thousand times.

23 We published the results in *JAMA* in 2009 and a follow-up study in *Academic Medicine* in 2012. See H. B. Beckman et al., "The Impact of a Program in Mindful Communication on Primary Care Physicians," *Academic Medicine* 87(6) (2012): 1–5; and M. S. Krasner et al., "Association of an Educational Program in Mindful Communication with Burnout, Empathy, and Attitudes among Primary Care Physicians," *JAMA* 302(12) (2009): 1284–93.

24 We assessed their personalities using the NEO five-factor scale, the most widely used assessment of personality. See P. T. Costa and R. R. McCrae, "NEO PI-R: Professional Manual, Revised Neo Personality Inventory (NEO PI-R), and Neo Five-Factor Inventory (NEO-FFI)" (Odessa, FL: Psychological Assessment Resources, 1992); R. R. McCrae and P. T. Costa Jr., "Personality Trait Structure as a Human Universal," *American Psychologist* 52(5) (1997): 509–16.

25 A 2014 study at the University of Pennsylvania reaffirms that physicians find their relationships with patients to be the most meaningful and rewarding aspects of their work. The researchers asked students and residents to identify physicians who exemplified humanistic patient care. These physicians reported attitudes, such as humility, and habits, such as self-reflection and mindfulness practices, that contributed to their effectiveness as healers and a reduction in burnout. See C. M. Chou, K. Kellom, and J. A. Shea, "Attitudes and Habits of Highly Humanistic Physicians," *Academic Medicine* 89(9) (2014): 1252–58.

26 See A. Verghese, "Culture Shock—Patient as Icon, Icon as Patient," *New England Journal of Medicine* 359(26) (2008): 2748–51.

27 Initially, the concepts of population health and evidence-based medicine ignored individual patients' perspectives and needs or developed quantitative models to incorporate "values" into algorithms that would guide treatment. The limitations have fortunately been addressed in the more recent conceptualizations of evidence-based medicine, which now incorporate elements of patient-centeredness. See D. Bassler et al., "Evidence-Based Medicine Targets the Individual Patient. Part 2: Guides and Tools for Individual Decision-Making," *ACP Journal Club* 149(1) (2008): 2; V. M. Montori and G. H. Guyatt, "Progress in Evidence-Based Medicine," *JAMA* 300(15) (2008):

1814–16; and G. Guyatt et al., "Patients at the Center: In Our Practice, and in Our Use of Language," *ACP Journal Club* 140(1) (2004): A11–A12.

28 My personal experience has been with the Zen and the Vipassana meditation traditions. These and other contemplative practices have in common a moment-to-moment attention to one's experience, cultivation of focus, and/or receptiveness and a nonjudgmental attitude. For some, martial arts or running or playing music serve similar ends. The important features are dedication, consistency, perseverance, and a sense of community. See chapter 11 and the appendix for more details.

2. ATTENDING

1 This quote is attributed to the late (and great) American baseball hero and philosopher Yogi Berra.

2 Sadly, Emil did not do well. His oncologist assured us, though, that the outcome would have been the same even if he had been diagnosed a month earlier.

3 This observation is now the title of a bestselling book, *The Invisible Gorilla*, which explores the phenomenon in all of its depth. C. Chabris and D. Simons, *The Invisible Gorilla: How Our Intuitions Deceive Us* (New York: Crown, 2011). For one version of this video, see http://www.youtube.com/watch?v=47LCLoidJh4.

4 The gorilla is in the upper-right portion of the (black) lung fields. See T. Drew, M. L. Vo, and J. M. Wolfe, "The Invisible Gorilla Strikes Again: Sustained Inattentional Blindness in Expert Observers," *Psychological Science* 24(9) (2013): 1848–53.

5 I am not sure why others did not speak up. Perhaps they too did not notice, or were afraid of the surgeon's reactions.

6 J. S. Macdonald and N. Lavie, "Visual Perceptual Load Induces Inattentional Deafness," *Attention, Perception, and Psychophysics* 73(6) (2011): 1780–89.

7 D. Kahneman, *Thinking, Fast and Slow* (New York: Farrar, Straus and Giroux, 2013).

8 I thank David Leach, formerly the head of the Accreditation Council for Graduate Medical Education, for introducing me to this Aristotelian concept in the context of medical practice and the literature that supports it. To understand better how expertise is more than just being experienced, see C. Bereiter and M. Scardamalia, *Surpassing Ourselves: An Inquiry into the Nature and Implications of Expertise* (Chicago: Open Court, 1993).

9 W. Levinson, R. Gorawara-Bhat, and J. Lamb, "A Study of Patient Clues and Physician Responses in Primary Care and Surgical Settings," *JAMA* 284(8) (2000): 1021–27; and A. L. Suchman et al., "A Model of Empathic Communication in the Medical Interview," *JAMA* 277(8) (1997): 678–82.

10 D. S. Morse, E. A. Edwardsen, and H. S. Gordon, "Missed Opportunities for Interval Empathy in Lung Cancer Communication," *Archives of Internal Medicine* 168(17) (2008): 1853–58.

11 More about this later in the discussion about the contribution of emotions to decision making in chapter 6.

12 Physicians provided informed consent to participate in the study and agreed to see two "unannounced standardized patients" during the subsequent year. See R. M. Epstein et al., "'Could This Be Something Serious?' Reassurance, Uncertainty, and Empathy in Response to Patients' Expressions of Worry," *Journal of General Internal Medicine* 22(12) (2007): 1731–39; and D. B. Seaburn et al., "Physician Responses to Ambiguous Patient Symptoms," *Journal of General Internal Medicine* 20(6) (2005): 525–30.

13 R. M. Epstein et al., "Awkward Moments in Patient-Physician Communication about HIV Risk," *Annals of Internal Medicine* 128(6) (1998): 435–42.

14 One recent review of the influence of patient-clinician communication and relationships in clinical care is J. M. Kelley et al., "The Influence of the Patient-Clinician Relationship on Healthcare Outcomes: A Systematic Review and Meta-analysis of Randomized Controlled Trials," *PLoS ONE* 9(4) (2014).

15 R. J. Baron, "An Introduction to Medical Phenomenology: I Can't Hear You While I'm Listening," *Annals of Internal Medicine* 103(4) (1985): 606–11.

16 Philosopher Michael Polanyi coined the term *subsidiary awareness*, a prerequisite for the capacity to slow down when you should; and *attention in automaticity* was described by surgeon Carol-Anne Moulton and physician Annie Leung. See M. Polanyi, *The Tacit Dimension* (Gloucester, MA: Peter Smith, 1983); and A. S. O. Leung, R. M. Epstein, and C.-A. Moulton, "The Competent Mind: Beyond Cognition," in *The Question of Competence*, eds. B. D. Hodges and L. Lingard (Ithaca and London: Cornell University Press, 2012), chap. 7, 155–76.

17 D. D. Salvucci, N. A. Taatgen, and J. P. Borst, "Toward a Unified Theory of the Multitasking Continuum: From Concurrent Performance to Task Switching, Interruption, and Resumption," *Proceedings of ACM CHI 2009 Conference on Human Factors in Computing Systems—Understanding UI 2* (2009): 1819–28.

18 There is a large literature in education and psychology on the effects of manipulating extraneous cognitive load (that which is not related to the problem at hand) and germane cognitive load (that which is related) on problem-solving capacity. See J. Sweller, "Cognitive Load During Problem Solving: Effects on Learning," *Cognitive Science* 12(2) (1988): 257–85; N. W. Mulligan, "The Role of Attention during Encoding in Implicit and Explicit Memory," *Journal of Experimental Psychology: Learning, Memory, & Cognition* 21(1) (1998): 27–47; and C. Stangor and D. McMillan, "Memory for Expectancy-Congruent and Expectancy-Incongruent Information," *Psychological Bulletin* 111(1) (1992): 42–61. For a more nuanced understanding of how attitude and motivation can "undo" this effect and promote recognition of inconsistent data, see J. W. Sherman, F. R. Conrey, and C. J. Groom, "Encoding Flexibility Revisited: Evidence for Enhanced Encoding of Stereotype-Inconsistent Information under Cognitive Load," *Social Cognition* 22(2) (2004): 214–32.

19 For a more detailed exploration of top-down and bottom-up attention, see M. Corbetta and G. L. Shulman, "Control of Goal-Directed and Stimulus-Driven Attention in the Brain," *Nature Reviews Neuroscience* 3(3) (2002): 201–15.

20 Rashes are common in innocuous viral illnesses, but some kinds can signal something more serious—measles, meningitis, or severe medication reactions.

21 For a discussion of the structure and function of the right frontoparietal network, and the importance of the right-sided lateralization, see Corbetta and Shulman, "Control of Goal-Directed." The right-left hemispheric differences are oversimplifications often promoted by popularized neuroscience. Current research suggests there are more similarities in function than differences, yet clearly some dysfunction is localized. For example, depression is associated with overactivity of the right prefrontal cortex compared to the left; those who have had right-sided strokes tend to be oblivious of their deficits, etc.

22 See Bereiter and Scardamalia, *Surpassing Ourselves*.

23 Attending to everything important is not always possible or desirable at any given moment, especially in emergency situations.

24 Psychologists describe "change blindness," in which gradual or unexpected changes in an image go unrecognized. For examples of gradual change blindness, see http://www.youtube.com/watch?v=1nL5ulsWMYc.

25 Drug warnings occur an average of sixty-three times—one every eight to ten minutes—during a typical physician's workday. See A. L. Russ et al., "Prescribers' Interactions with Medication Alerts at the Point of Prescribing: A Multi-method, In Situ Investigation of the Human-Computer Interaction," *International Journal of Medical Informatics* 81(4) (2012): 232–43.

26 The original source is K. Maue, *Water in the Lake: Real Events for the Imagination* (New York: Harper & Row, 1979). Ken Maue taught at Wesleyan University in the 1970s, and his brilliant ways of bringing awareness to the ordinary were stunning. A musician by training, his avant-garde "pieces" became gradually less concerned with sound and more about how we can experience any environment as "music." His pieces reveal our inner lives in ways similar to those of formal contemplative practice—they sculpt our capacity for awareness.

27 The idea of immaculate perception is hardly original. The concept had its origins in both Western and Buddhist philosophy, later to be confirmed with empirical studies. Buddhist philosophy emphasizes both the emptiness of all things including perceptions, and that through meditation one can strip away meaning, judgment, and bias, permitting us to see the world as it is. See F. J. Streng, *Emptiness: A Study in Religious Meaning* (Nashville, TN: Abingdon Press, 1967). Francis Bacon (1605) asserted that immaculate perception was necessary to see the world as it is, "keeping the eye steadily fixed upon the facts of nature and so receiving the images simply as they are." Nietzsche, in *Thus Spake Zarathustra*, refuted that this would be possible, given that we have desires and wishes that will color our perceptions. Author Anaïs Nin reflected this sentiment in her oft-quoted passage on how we "do not see things as they are, we see them as we are." See A. Nin, *The Diary of Anaïs Nin, 1939–1944* (New York: Harcourt, Brace & World, 1969). The lack of immaculate perception has repeatedly been established in social psychology using studies of implicit (unconscious) bias and stereotyping, as noted in T. D. Wilson, *Strangers to Ourselves: Discovering the Adaptive Unconscious* (Cambridge, MA: Belknap Press of Harvard Universtiy Press, 2002). In medicine, these biases have been shown to influence clinical decisions. See A. R. Green et al., "Implicit Bias among Physicians and Its Prediction

of Thrombolysis Decisions for Black and White Patients," *Journal of General Internal Medicine* 22(9) (2007): 1231–38. A TEDx Talk by Jerry Kang exhibits this principle clearly: http://thesituationist.wordpress.com/2014/02/01/immaculate-perception. In this book, I propose that it is possible, through self-awareness, to access some of these processes that are normally below the level of awareness.

28 Scripts are internalized mental stories based on prototypical clinical scenarios—often learned during training. See B. Charlin et al., "Scripts and Clinical Reasoning," *Medical Education* 41(12) (2007): 1178–84.

29 Patrick Croskerry, a Canadian emergency-medicine physician, describes "cognitive dispositions to respond," intrinsic biases that affect clinical decision making. They are described well in J. E. Groopman, *How Doctors Think* (New York: Houghton Mifflin, 2007). Croskerry outlines dozens of sources of bias, stereotyping, and misapplied heuristics in a series of articles over the past fifteen years, from misplaced attribution, overconfidence, and premature closure. Most of these processes are below the level of awareness. For further reading, see P. Croskerry and G. Norman, "Overconfidence in Clinical Decision Making," *American Journal of Medicine* 121(5) (2008): S24–S29; P. Croskerry and G. R. Nimmo, "Better Clinical Decision Making and Reducing Diagnostic Error," *Journal of the Royal College of Physicians of Edinburgh* 41(2) (2011): 155–62; P. Croskerry, A. A. Abbass, and A. W. Wu, "How Doctors Feel: Affective Issues in Patients' Safety," *Lancet* 372(9645) (2008): 1205–6; P. Croskerry, "The Importance of Cognitive Errors in Diagnosis and Strategies to Minimize Them," *Academic Medicine* 78(8) (2003): 775–80; P. Croskerry, "Clinical Cognition and Diagnostic Error: Applications of a Dual Process Model of Reasoning," *Advances in Health Sciences Education* 14(1) (2009): 27–35; and P. Croskerry, "From Mindless to Mindful Practice—Cognitive Bias and Clinical Decision Making," *New England Journal of Medicine* 368(26) (2013): 2445–48.

30 A series of laboratory experiments confirming these observations were done by Mohanty's lab. See A. Mohanty et al., "Search for a Threatening Target Triggers Limbic Guidance of Spatial Attention," *Journal of Neuorscience* 29(34) (2009): 10563–72; and A. Mohanty and T. J. Sussman, "Top-Down Modulation of Attention by Emotion," *Frontiers in Human Neuroscience* 7 (2013): 102.

31 Stereotyping in medicine clearly goes beyond individual patient behaviors and includes race, ethnicity, gender, sexual orientation, habits, obesity, lifestyle choices, and diseases, which I'll discuss in greater detail later in the book.

32 The dermatologist Neil Prose describes a similar situation, in which a patient's psychological distress was only apparent after he looked deeper than her skin. See N. Prose, "Paying Attention," *JAMA* 283(21) (2000): 2763.

33 Carol-Anne Moulton calls this quality "attention in automaticity." See C.-A. Moulton et al., "Slowing Down When You Should: A New Model of Expert Judgment," *Academic Medicine RIME: Proceedings of the Forty-Sixth Annual Conference* 82(10) (2007): S109–S116.

3. CURIOSITY

1 Some of the content of this chapter is drawn from an article I wrote with Larry Dyche: L. Dyche and R. M. Epstein, "Curiosity and Medical Education," *Medical Education* 45(7) (2011): 663–68. Also see D. E. Berlyne, "Novelty and Curiosity as Determinants of Exploratory Behaviour," *British Journal of Psychiatry* 41(1–2) (1950): 68–80.

2 From Erich Leowy, quoted in F. T. Fitzgerald, "Curiosity," *Annals of Internal Medicine* 130(1) (1999): 70–72.

3 Here I'm referring to the five-factor model of personality. See R. R. McCrae et al., "Nature over Nurture: Temperament, Personality, and Life Span Development," *Journal of Personality and Social Psychology* 78(1) (2000): 173–86.

4 Uncertainty in medicine and physicians' reactions to uncertainty have been explored in depth since Renee Fox's seminal 1959 book. Here is a selection of perspectives, but space does not allow inclusion of a comprehensive set of references: R. Fox, *Experiment Perilous: Physicians and Patients Facing the Unknown* (Glencoe, IL: Free Press, 1959); J. P. Kassirer, "Our Stubborn Quest for Diagnostic Certainty: A Cause of Excessive Testing," *New England Journal of Medicine* 320(22) (1989): 1489–91; F. Borrell-Carrió and R. M. Epstein, "Preventing Errors in Clinical Practice: A Call for Self-Awareness," *Annals of Family Medicine* 2(4) (2004): 310–16; G. Gillett, "Clinical Medicine and the Quest for Certainty," *Social Science & Medicine* 58(4) (2004): 727–38; K. G. Volz and G. Gigerenzer, "Cognitive Processes in Decisions under Risk Are Not the Same as in Decisions under Uncertainty," *Frontiers in Decision Neuroscience* 6(105) (2012): 1–6; R. M. Epstein, B. S. Alper, and T. E. Quill, "Communicating Evidence for Participatory Decision Making," *JAMA* 291(19) (2004): 2359–66; R. M. Epstein et al., "'Could This Be Something Serious?' Reassurance, Uncertainty, and Empathy in Response to Patients' Expressions of Worry," *Journal of General Internal Medicine* 22(12) (2007): 1731–39; M. S. Gerrity, R. F. DeVellis, and J. A. Earp, "Physicians' Reactions to Uncertainty in Patient Care: A New Measure and New Insights," *Medical Care* 28(8) (1990): 724–36; G. H. Gordon, S. K. Joos, and J. Byrne, "Physician Expressions of Uncertainty during Patient Encounters," *Patient Education & Counseling* 40(1) (2000): 59–65; C. G. Johnson et al., "Does Physician Uncertainty Affect Patient Satisfaction?," *Journal of General Internal Medicine* 3(2) (1988): 144–49; and J. Ogden et al., "Doctors' Expressions of Uncertainty and Patient Confidence," *Patient Education & Counseling* 48(2) (2002): 171–76.

5 Fitzgerald, "Curiosity."

6 In 1912 the *Titanic* hit an iceberg on its maiden voyage, killing the majority of those on board.

7 Just out of curiosity, I checked my own medical chart. There were thirty problems listed, most of which had resolved decades ago. Only two were actually relevant to my current health.

8 E. Baumgarten, "Curiosity as a Moral Virtue," *International Journal of Applied Philosophy* 15(2) (2001): 23–42; J. Halpern, *From Detached Concern to Empathy: Humanizing Medical Practice* (Oxford: Oxford Univer-

sity Press, 2001); Institute of Medicine, *Crossing the Quality Chasm: A New Health System for the 21st Century* (Washington, DC: National Academies Press, 2001); R. M. Epstein et al., "Measuring Patient-Centered Communication in Patient-Physician Consultations: Theoretical and Practical Issues," *Social Science & Medicine* 61(7) (2005): 1516–28; and C. M. Chou, K. Kellom, and J. A. Shea, "Attitudes and Habits of Highly Humanistic Physicians," *Academic Medicine* 89(9) (2014): 1252–58.

9 See M. Polanyi, "Knowing and Being, the Logic of Tacit Inference," in *Knowing and Being: Essays by Michael Polanyi*, ed. M. Grene (Chicago: University of Chicago Press, 1969), chaps. 9 and 10, 123–58; and M. Polanyi, *Personal Knowledge: Towards a Post-critical Philosophy* (Chicago: University of Chicago Press, 1974).

10 V. F. Reyna, "A Theory of Medical Decision Making and Health: Fuzzy Trace Theory," *Medical Decision Making* 28(6) (2008): 850–65.

11 For interesting discussions about informed intuition in expert practice, see M. C. Price, "Intuitive Decisions on the Fringes of Consciousness: Are They Conscious and Does It Matter?," *Judgment and Decision Making* 3(1) (2008): 28–41; V. F. Reyna and F. J. Lloyd, "Physician Decision Making and Cardiac Risk: Effects of Knowledge, Risk Perception, Risk Tolerance, and Fuzzy Processing," *Journal of Experimental Psychology: Applied* 12(3) (2006): 179; and D. Kahneman and G. Klein, "Conditions for Intuitive Expertise: A Failure to Disagree," *American Psychologist* 64(6) (2009): 515–26.

12 The body scan can be done lying down or sitting, or even standing. The instructions are simple, and guided body scans are readily available on the Web if you want to try it yourself. An audio-recorded guided body scan can be accessed at http://www.urmc.rochester.edu/family-medicine/mindful -practice/curricula-materials/audios.aspx.

13 Thanks to Laura Hogan for this story.

14 E. J. Langer, *The Power of Mindful Learning* (Reading, MA: Perseus Books, 1997); and G. C. Spivak, L. E. Lyons, and C. G. Franklin, "'On the Cusp of the Personal and the Impersonal': An Interview with Gayatri Chakravorty Spivak," *Biography* 27(1) (2004): 203–21.

15 More about doubt and uncertainty in chapters 4 and 6.

16 J. Greenberg and N. Meiran, "Is Mindfulness Meditation Associated with 'Feeling Less'?," *Mindfulness* 5(5) (2014): 471–76.

17 C. R. Horowitz et al., "What Do Doctors Find Meaningful about Their Work?," *Annals of Internal Medicine* 138(9) (2003): 772–75.

18 See T. B. Kashdan et al., "Curiosity Enhances the Role of Mindfulness in Reducing Defensive Responses to Existential Threat," *Personality and Individual Differences* 50(8) (2011): 1227–32; and C. P. Niemiec et al., "Being Present in the Face of Existential Threat: The Role of Trait Mindfulness in Reducing Defensive Responses to Mortality Salience," *Journal of Personality and Social Psychology* 99(2) (2010): 344–65.

19 C. Kidd and B. Y. Hayden, "The Psychology and Neuroscience of Curiosity," *Neuron* 88(3) (2015): 449–60.

20 J. Gottlieb et al., "Information-Seeking, Curiosity, and Attention: Computational and Neural Mechanisms," *Trends in Cognitive Sciences* 17(11) (2013): 585–93.

21 Dopamine drives exploration behaviors in humans and animals and also affects memory and intelligence. In the prefrontal cortex, which processes executive decision making, impulse control, and other cognitive processes, one particular dopamine receptor is strongly expressed, the D4 receptor. Catechol-O-methyltransferase is an enzyme that breaks down dopamine and other neurotransmitters and is also active in the prefrontal cortex. Thus, the current model is that both genes for dopamine D4 receptor and COMT may affect curiosity. R. P. Ebstein et al., "Dopamine D4 Receptor (D4DR) Exon III Polymorphism Associated with the Human Personality Trait of Novelty Seeking," *Nature Genetics* 12(1) (1996): 78–80; and C. G. DeYoung et al., "Sources of Cognitive Exploration: Genetic Variation in the Prefrontal Dopamine System Predicts Openness/Intellect," *Journal of Research in Personality* 45(4) (2011): 364–71.

22 Here, and everywhere in this book, I apologize for the oversimplifications of complex multidimensional biological processes with complex control mechanisms that have been coalesced into pathways for heuristic value, but diminish the marvel of their interconnections. In particular, social epigenetics is in its infancy as an area of scientific pursuit, and while the basic principles—that the social environment affects gene expression—will prove enduring, the details of how this happens will undoubtedly undergo radical revisions.

23 Dyche and Epstein, "Curiosity and Medical Education"; and L. K. Michaelson, A. B. Knight, and D. Flink, *Team-Based Learning: A Transformative Use of Small Groups* (New York: Praeger Publishing, 2002).

24 P. Fonagy et al., *Affect Regulation, Mentalization, and the Development of Self* (New York: Other Press, 2002); and D. W. Winnicott, *The Maturational Processes and the Facilitating Environment* (Madison, CT: International Universities Press, 1965).

25 E. J. Langer, *Mindfulness* (Reading, MA: Addison-Wesley, 1989); Langer, *Power of Mindful Learning*; D. A. Schon, *The Reflective Practitioner* (New York: Basic Books, 1983); N. H. Leonard and M. Harvey, "Curiosity, Mindfulness and Learning Style in the Acquisition of Knowledge by Individuals/Organisations," *International Journal of Learning and Intellectual Capital* 4(3) (2007): 294–314; J. P. Fry, "Interactive Relationship between Inquisitiveness and Student Control of Instruction," *Journal of Educational Psychology* 68(5) (1972): 459–65; and B. Roman and J. Kay, "Fostering Curiosity: Using the Educator-Learner Relationship to Promote a Facilitative Learning Environment," *Psychiatry: Interpersonal and Biological Processes* 70(3) (2007): 205–8.

26 Strong attachment to friends and family during adulthood influences curiosity and exploration in the work environment. Those whose work environments are unsupportive, though, are forced to derive support exclusively from their relationships with family and friends. However, family and friends quickly tire of medical talk and the difficult situations that doctors face. See A. J. Elliot and H. T. Reis, "Attachment and Exploration in Adulthood," *Journal of Personality and Social Psychology* 85(2) (2003): 317–31.

27 E. R. Kandel, "A New Intellectual Framework for Psychiatry," *American Journal of Psychiatry* 155(4) (1998): 457–69.

4. BEGINNER'S MIND

1 S. Suzuki, *Zen Mind, Beginner's Mind* (New York: Weatherhill, 1980).

2 Suzuki Roshi died three years before I arrived in San Francisco, yet his teachings about beginner's mind were and remain guideposts of practice at the center.

3 Stewart and Hubert Dreyfus observed chess players and professionals in a variety of fields to understand how experts get that way. They developed a model of a hierarchy from novice, advanced beginner, competent, proficient, and expert, only later adding a level for master. See H. L. Dreyfus, *On the Internet (Thinking in Action)* (New York: Routledge, 2001).

4 C. G. Shields et al., "Pain Assessment: The Roles of Physician Certainty and Curiosity," *Health Communication* 28(7) (2013): 740–46.

5 M. Hojat et al., "The Devil Is in the Third Year: A Longitudinal Study of Erosion of Empathy in Medical School," *Academic Medicine* 84(9) (2009): 1182–91.

6 A series of neuroimaging studies conducted by a research group in Taiwan provides some clues as to how this happens. The researchers prepared a set of brief videos in which one set of actors was touched by Q-tips and another set underwent acupuncture. They showed the videos to doctors who practice acupuncture. The control group was nonclinicians, matched for age and educational level. The brain activity of both doctors and nonclinicians was monitored using a variety of functional neuroimaging techniques (initially MRI scanning, with follow-up studies using magnetoencephalography and electroencephalography) to demonstrate how doctors' expertise modulates how they perceive the pain of others. Among nonexperts, witnessing a patient undergoing acupuncture (as compared to being touched by a Q-tip) produced responses in the sensory and emotion-processing parts of the brain, reflecting some degree of emotional resonance and empathy. However, among physician-acupuncturists, those areas were deactivated, and instead, other areas of the brain were activated—particularly those involved in regulating emotions and a cognitive understanding of (but not emotional resonance with) the patient's experience (so-called theory of mind); their growing expertise leads them to see the world differently. This ability—to regulate emotions and categorize illness into disease categories—is fundamental to good care. Yet, there is an unnecessary imbalance, and it doesn't have to be that way—we can have both technical expertise and human understanding. See J. Decety, C. Y. Yang, and Y. Cheng, "Physicians Down-Regulate Their Pain Empathy Response: An Event-Related Brain Potential Study," *NeuroImage* 50(4) (2010): 1676–82; and Y. Cheng et al., "The Perception of Pain in Others Suppresses Somatosensory Oscillations: A Magnetoencephalography Study," *NeuroImage* 40(4) (2008): 1833–40.

7 P. Goldberg, *The Intuitive Edge: Understanding and Developing Intuition* (Los Angeles: J. P. Tarcher, 1983).

8 Karl Ditters von Dittersdorf was a well-respected eighteenth-century composer, whose music is faultless but clearly without the inspiration of Haydn, Mozart, or Bach.

9 P. Croskerry, "From Mindless to Mindful Practice—Cognitive Bias and Clinical Decision Making," *New England Journal of Medicine* 368(26) (2013): 2445–48.

10 The source is F. S. Fitzgerald, "The Crack Up," in *The Crack Up*, ed. E. Wilson (New York: New Directions, 1945). However, the idea is not new. The poet John Keats considered creativity to spring from the rejection of constraining philosophies and absolute truths and the seeking of mystery and doubt. Keats influenced pragmatist philosophers such as John Dewey, and perhaps also Fitzgerald.

11 While this quote has been attributed to Einstein, the source has never been found and many others have made similar observations.

12 This Zen story is quoted in many sources, originally from a Zen classic now in translation as K. Yamada, *The Gateless Gate: The Classic Book of Zen Koans* (New York: Simon & Schuster, 2005).

13 From a talk by G. Fronsdal, "Not-Knowing," http://www.insightmeditation center.org/books-articles/articles/not-knowing.

14 L. Festinger, "Cognitive Dissonance," *Scientific American* 207(4) (1962): 93–107.

15 The many ways in which physicians can deceive themselves during diagnoses is explored in J. E. Groopman, *How Doctors Think* (New York: Houghton Mifflin, 2007).

16 G. E. Simon and O. Gureje, "Stability of Somatization Disorder and Somatization Symptoms among Primary Care Patients," *Archives of General Psychiatry* 56(1) (1999): 90–95.

17 This story has multiple sources, including P. Reps and N. Senzaki, *Zen Flesh, Zen Bones: A Collection of Zen and Pre-Zen Writings* (Clarendon, VT: Tuttle Publishing, 1998).

18 D. J. Levitin, *The Organized Mind: Thinking Straight in the Age of Information Overload* (New York: Dutton Adult, 2014); Croskerry, "From Mindless to Mindful Practice"; P. Croskerry and G. Norman, "Overconfidence in Clinical Decision Making," *American Journal of Medicine* 121(5) (2008): S24–S29; and P. Croskerry, "The Importance of Cognitive Errors in Diagnosis and Strategies to Minimize Them," *Academic Medicine* 78(8) (2003): 775–80.

19 J. Dewey, *Experience and Nature* (New York: Dover, 1958).

20 For an eloquent discussion of fragile categories and their philosophical and pragmatic implications, see W. James, *Pragmatism* (Cambridge, MA: Harvard University Press, 1975). For a Buddhist perspective on the emptiness of categories, see F. J. Streng, *Emptiness: A Study in Religious Meaning* (Nashville, TN: Abingdon Press, 1967).

21 C. Barks, *The Essential Rumi* (London: Castle Books, 1997).

22 G. Norman, M. Young, and L. Brooks, "Non-analytical Models of Clinical Reasoning: The Role of Experience," *Medical Education* 41(12) (2007): 1140–45.

23 See T. J. Kaptchuk, *The Web That Has No Weaver: Understanding Chinese Medicine* (New York: Congdon & Weed, 1983).

24 See J. Greenberg, K. Reiner, and N. Meiran, "'Mind the Trap': Mindfulness Practice Reduces Cognitive Rigidity," *PLoS ONE* 7(5) (2012): e36206.

25 This intervention had many of the same elements as our physician training programs.

26 See J. Connelly, "Being in the Present Moment: Developing the Capacity for Mindfulness in Medicine," *Academic Medicine* 74(4) (1999): 420–24.

27 D. A. Schön, *Educating the Reflective Practitioner* (San Francisco: Jossey-Bass, 1987).

5. BEING PRESENT

1 Philosopher Michel Foucault described how a "clinical gaze," in contrast to usual social interactions, objectifies and disempowers patients, especially in hospital settings. See M. Foucault, *The Birth of the Clinic: An Archaeology of Medical Perception* (New York: Random House, 1994). Philosopher Emmanuel Levinas describes how ethical behavior starts with apprehending another's face, more so than principles, words, and ideas. For further discussion of Levinas's ethical mandate of immediacy in health care contexts, see R. Naef, "Bearing Witness: A Moral Way of Engaging in the Nurse-Person Relationship," *Nursing Philosophy* 7(3) (2006): 146–56; P. Komesaroff, "The Many Faces of the Clinic: A Levinasian View," in *Handbook of Phenomenology and Medicine*, ed. S. K. Toombs (Dordrecht, Netherlands: Kluwer Academic Publishers, 2001), 317–30; and J. V. Welie, "Towards an Ethics of Immediacy: A Defense of a Noncontractual Foundation of the Care Giver–Patient Relationship," *Medicine, Health Care, and Philosophy* 2(1) (1999): 11–19.

2 A. L. Suchman and D. A. Matthews, "What Makes the Patient-Doctor Relationship Therapeutic? Exploring the Connexional Dimension of Medical Care," *Annals of Internal Medicine* 108(1) (1988): 125–30.

3 M. K. Marvel et al., "Soliciting the Patient's Agenda: Have We Improved?," *JAMA* 281(3) (1999): 283–87.

4 I am grateful to Steve McPhee, M.D., who generously shared with me his thoughts on presence and his inspiration by the works of Harper and Marcel. See R. Harper, *On Presence: Variations and Reflections* (Philadelphia: Trinity Press International, 1991).

5 The idea of an observing self has been approached from educational, psychoanalytic, philosophical, and, more recently, neuroscientific perspectives. Here are some entry points into a rich literature: M. Epstein, *Thoughts without a Thinker: Psychotherapy from a Buddhist Perspective* (New York: Basic Books, 1995); R. M. Epstein, D. J. Siegel, and J. Silberman, "Self-Monitoring in Clinical Practice: A Challenge for Medical Educators," *Journal of Continuing Education in the Health Professions* 28(1) (2008): 5–13; and B. J. Baars, T. Z. Ramsoy, and S. Laureys, "Brain, Conscious Experience and the Observing Self," *Trends in Neurosciences* 26(12) (2003): 671–75.

6 J. E. Connelly, "Narrative Possibilities: Using Mindfulness in Clinical Practice," *Perspectives in Biology and Medicine* 48(1) (2005): 84–94; J. Coulehan, "Compassionate Solidarity: Suffering, Poetry, and Medicine," *Perspectives in Biology and Medicine* 52(4) (2009): 585–603; J. L. Coulehan, "Tenderness and Steadiness: Emotions in Medical Practice," *Literature and Medicine* 14(2)

(1995): 222–36; and R. Charon, "Narrative Medicine: Form, Function, and Ethics," *Annals of Internal Medicine* 134(1) (2001): 83–87.

7 This story is discussed in an article and cited with permission in R. M. Epstein, "Making the Ineffable Visible," *Families, Systems, & Health* 33(3) (2015): 280–82.

8 K. J. Swayden et al., "Effect of Sitting vs. Standing on Perception of Provider Time at Bedside: A Pilot Study," *Patient Education & Counseling* 86(2) (2012): 166–71.

9 K. Zoppi, "Communication about Concerns in Well-Child Visits" (Ann Arbor: University of Michigan, 1994).

10 A. L. Back et al., "Compassionate Silence in the Patient-Clinician Encounter: A Contemplative Approach," *Journal of Palliative Medicine* 12(12) (2009): 1113–17; and J. Bartels et al., "Eloquent Silences: A Musical and Lexical Analysis of Conversation between Oncologists and Their Patients," *Patient Education & Counseling* (forthcoming, 2016).

11 C. Lamm, C. D. Batson, and J. Decety, "The Neural Substrate of Human Empathy: Effects of Perspective-Taking and Cognitive Appraisal," *Journal of Cognitive Neuroscience* 19(1) (2007): 42–58.

12 C. Barks, *The Essential Rumi* (London: Castle Books, 1997); and J. E. Connelly, "The Guest House (Commentary)," *Academic Medicine* 83(6) (2008): 588–89.

13 G. Riva et al., "From Intention to Action: The Role of Presence," *New Ideas in Psychology* 29(1) (2011): 24–37.

14 J. Leff et al., "Computer-Assisted Therapy for Medication-Resistant Auditory Hallucinations: Proof-of-Concept Study," *British Journal of Psychiatry* 202(6) (2013): 428–33.

15 This understanding—that the mind is relational—is a radical departure from earlier notions of how the mind works. Giuseppe Riva and philosopher Evan Thompson and neuroscientist Antonio Damasio all suggest—from very different philosophical points of view—that "mind" emerges as a property of the relationship among a brain, a body, and the world, and from that embodied extended mind a sense of self and a sense of presence emerge.

16 See E. Thompson and M. Stapleton, "Making Sense of Sense-Making: Reflections on Enactive and Extended Mind Theories," *Topoi* 28(1) (2009): 23–30.

17 To understand more about intersubjectivity, I'd suggest starting with M. Buber, *I and Thou* (New York: Scribner, 1970); and N. Pembroke, "Human Dimension in Medical Care: Insights from Buber and Marcel," *Southern Medical Journal* 103(12) (2010): 1210–13.

18 As I've mentioned before, this skill "works" only if one has the ability to maintain enough differentiation between oneself and the other person to understand which experiences are yours and which are the other's—otherwise it disintegrates into shared delusion.

19 D. B. Baker, R. Day, and E. Salas, "Teamwork as an Essential Component of High-Reliability Organizations," *Health Services Research* 41(4, pt. 2) (2006): 1576–98.

20 J. Chatel-Goldman et al., "Non-local Mind from the Perspective of Social Cognition," *Frontiers in Human Neuroscience* 7 (2013): 107; and J. Zlatev et

al., "Intersubjectivity: What Makes Us Human?," in *The Shared Mind: Perspectives on Intersubjectivity*, eds. J. Zlatev, T. P. Racine, C. Sinha, and E. Itkonen (Amsterdam and Philadelphia: John Benjamins, 2008), chap. 1, 1–14.

21 W. B. Ventres and R. M. Frankel, "Shared Presence in Physician-Patient Communication: A Graphic Representation," *Families, Systems, & Health* 33(3) (2015): 270–79.

22 See R. Klitzman, *When Doctors Become Patients* (New York: Oxford University Press, 2008).

23 Dozens of studies document implicit bias in health care. Here are a few: D. J. Burgess, "Are Providers More Likely to Contribute to Healthcare Disparities under High Levels of Cognitive Load? How Features of the Healthcare Setting May Lead to Biases in Medical Decision Making," *Medical Decision Making* 30(2) (2010): 246–57; J. A. Sabin, F. P. Rivara, and A. G. Greenwald, "Physician Implicit Attitudes and Stereotypes about Race and Quality of Medical Care," *Medical Care* 46(7) (2008): 678–85; D. J. Burgess, S. S. Fu, and M. van Ryn, "Why Do Providers Contribute to Disparities and What Can Be Done About It?," *Journal of General Internal Medicine* 19(11) (2004): 1154–59; M. van Ryn, "Research on the Provider Contribution to Race/Ethnicity Disparities in Medical Care," *MedCare* 40(1) (2002): I140–I151; and J. Sabin et al., "Physicians' Implicit and Explicit Attitudes about Race by MD Race, Ethnicity, and Gender," *Journal of Health Care for the Poor and Underserved* 20(3) (2009): 896–913.

24 W. J. Hall et al., "Implicit Racial/Ethnic Bias among Health Care Professionals and Its Influence on Health Care Outcomes: A Systematic Review," *American Journal of Public Health* 105(12) (2015): e60–e76.

25 R. M. Epstein et al., "Understanding Fear of Contagion among Physicians Who Care for HIV Patients," *Family Medicine* 25(4) (1993): 264–68; and J. Shapiro, "Walking a Mile in Their Patients' Shoes: Empathy and Othering in Medical Students' Education," *Philosophy, Ethics, and Humanities in Medicine* 3(1) (2008): 1.

26 J. A. Bartz et al., "Oxytocin Selectively Improves Empathic Accuracy," *Psychological Science* 21(10) (2010): 1426–28; and C. K. De Dreu, "Oxytocin Modulates Cooperation within and Competition between Groups: An Integrative Review and Research Agenda," *Hormones and Behavior* 61(3) (2012): 419–28.

27 For an interesting discussion of tribalism in modern culture, see J. Greene, *Moral Tribes: Emotion, Reason, and the Gap between Us and Them* (New York: Penguin Press, 2013).

28 With training, people can experience greater emotional resonance. As tribal beings, though, we squelch the resonance if we label the other person as "not like me." To make matters worse, the tendency to stereotype—and therefore distance—worsens when people are under high cognitive load, such as in the emergency room. T. J. Allen et al., "Stereotype Strength and Attentional Bias: Preference for Confirming versus Disconfirming Information Depends on Processing Capacity," *Journal of Experimental Social Psychology* 45(5) (2009): 1081–87; Burgess, "Are Providers More Likely to Contribute?"; and Burgess, Fu, and van Ryn, "Why Do Providers Contribute to Disparities?" An often-

quoted study by Knox Todd examined prescriptions for pain medications in a busy Los Angeles emergency room prescribed for Latinos and non-Latinos with long-bone fractures of equivalent severity. Latinos received far fewer prescriptions and for lower doses, and twice as many Latinos as Anglos received no pain medication at all: K. H. Todd, N. Samaroo, and J. R. Hoffman, "Ethnicity as a Risk Factor for Inadequate Emergency Department Analgesia," *JAMA* 269(12) (1993): 1537–39. Perhaps the physicians unconsciously viewed Latino patients as more stoic or that they were more likely to abuse medications. I'm not sure why and the study didn't ask. Cognitive load and unexamined bias surely had something to do with it. Bias is not restricted to ethnicity. Physicians use fewer tests for heart disease in women and blacks compared to white males with equivalent risk factors—K. A. Schulman et al., "The Effect of Race and Sex on Physicians' Recommendations for Cardiac Catheterization," *New England Journal of Medicine* 340(8) (1999): 618–26—and provide less adequate breast cancer treatments to black women as compared to white women with the same disease characteristics: V. L. Shavers and M. L. Brown, "Racial and Ethnic Disparities in the Receipt of Cancer Treatment," *Journal of the National Cancer Institute* 94(5) (2002): 334–57. Similar biases exist for patients who are overweight and of low educational level.

Bias is not acceptable for doctors and other professionals; our mandate is to serve everyone, including patients whose life experiences are vastly different from our own. Because people generally disavow bias, the first, and challenging, step is awareness. A somewhat controversial and fascinating test for measuring implicit biases—biases that are below the level of awareness—was developed using computer technology that measures how long you take to respond to questions associating race, for example, with positive and negative words. Called the implicit-association test, the scores correlate with our judgments about people's character, abilities, and potential. A free version can be found at https://implicit.harvard.edu/implicit/takeatest.html. For a good read about the test and its implications, see M. Banaji and A. Greenwald, *Blindspot: Hidden Biases of Good People* (New York: Delacorte Press, 2013). Also see J. F. Dovidio et al., "On the Nature of Prejudice: Automatic and Controlled Processes," *Journal of Experimental Social Psychology* 33(5) (1997): 510–40; and A. G. Greenwald, D. E. McGhee, and J. L. K. Schwartz, "Measuring Individual Differences in Implicit Cognition: The Implicit Association Test," *Journal of Personality and Social Psychology* 74(6) (1998): 1464–80. For example, a well-meaning and otherwise excellent doctor might believe that he treats men's and women's pain similarly, but the way he associates pain with gender during the test may reveal biases of which he is unaware and that influence his prescribing practices. People's reactions to the IAT range from bland acceptance to vehement denial; those who deny their biases, not surprisingly, have fewer means for accommodating and diminishing the effects of bias.

29 Specifically the areas of the brain that involve self-other differentiation and cognitive appraisal (i.e., the dorsomedial prefrontal cortex and right inferior frontal cortex). Social neuroscientists Claus Lamm and Jean Decety have demonstrated changes on functional MRI scans when people make the effort to appreciate the pain of those who are not like them. See C. Lamm, A. N.

Meltzoff, and J. Decety, "How Do We Empathize with Someone Who Is Not Like Us? A Functional Magnetic Resonance Imaging Study," *Journal of Cognitive Neuroscience* 22(2) (2010): 362–76.

30 J. Decety, C. Yang, and Y. Cheng, "Physicians Down-Regulate Their Pain Empathy Response: An Event-Related Brain Potential Study," *NeuroImage* 50(4) (2010): 1676–82.

31 R. L. Reniers et al., "Empathy, ToM, and Self-Other Differentiation: An fMRI Study of Internal States," *Social Neuroscience* 9(1) (2014): 50–62; and Lamm, Batson, Decety, "Neural Substrate of Human Empathy."

32 P. Fonagy et al., *Affect Regulation, Mentalization, and the Development of Self* (New York: Other Press, 2002).

33 See the discussion of social epigenetics in chapter 3, "Curiosity."

34 A. Lutz et al., "Bold Signal in Insula Is Differentially Related to Cardiac Function during Compassion Meditation in Experts vs. Novices," *NeuroImage* 47(3) (2009): 1038–46.

35 Evan Thompson and other cognitive scientists and philosophers have called this embodied cognition, or embodied mind. F. J. Varela, E. Thompson, and E. Rosch, *The Embodied Mind: Cognitive Science and Human Experience* (Cambridge, MA: MIT Press, 1991).

36 Cognitive science has finally caught up with millennia of experience with contemplative practices, helping us to understand, from a scientific standpoint, the connection between awareness of our physical selves and awareness of our thoughts and emotions—that first we experience the smile, then identify the emotion of happiness. A. R. Damasio. *The Feeling of What Happens: Body and Emotion in the Making of Consciousness* (New York: Harcourt Brace, 1999).

37 C.-M. Tan, *Search Inside Yourself* (New York: HarperCollins, 2012). Reprinted from https://siyli.org/two-siyli-ways-to-change-your-mind-2.

6. NAVIGATING WITHOUT A MAP

1 R. A. Rodenbach et al., "Relationships between Personal Attitudes about Death and Communication with Terminally Ill Patients: How Oncology Clinicians Grapple with Mortality," *Patient Education & Counseling* 99(3) (2015): 356–63.

2 The idea that people left to decide for themselves is not always autonomy-supportive and can actually undermine a sense of self-determination was proposed in S. Sherwin, *No Longer Patient: Feminist Ethics and Health Care* (Philadelphia: Temple University Press, 1992).

3 E. B. Larson and X. Yao, "Clinical Empathy as Emotional Labor in the Patient-Physician Relationship," *JAMA* 293(9) (2005): 1100–1106.

4 See J. R. Adams et al., "Communicating with Physicians about Medical Decisions: A Reluctance to Disagree," *Archives of Internal Medicine* 172(15) (2012): 1184–86.

5 S. Glouberman and B. Zimmerman, "Complicated and Complex Systems: What Would Successful Reform of Medicare Look Like?," in *Romanow*

Papers: Changing Health Care in Canada, eds. P.-G. Forest, G. P. Marchildon, and T. McIntosh (Toronto: University of Toronto Press, 2002).

6 Here decision aids for patients that include values checklists, informational videos, and patient testimonials can be helpful. See G. Elwyn et al., "Developing a Quality Criteria Framework for Patient Decision Aids: Online International Delphi Consensus Process," *BMJ* 333(7565) (2006): 417.

7 See T. E. Quill and H. Brody, "Physician Recommendations and Patient Autonomy: Finding a Balance between Physician Power and Patient Choice," *Annals of Internal Medicine* 125(9) (1996): 763–69. Also, for reasons I explored in chapter 4, physicians sometimes recommend treatments that they would not choose for themselves. See D. Gorenstein, "How Doctors Die: Showing Others the Way," *New York Times*, November 19, 2013, http://www.nytimes.com/2013/11/20/your-money/how-doctors-die.html?_r=2.

8 C. E. Lindblom, "The Science of 'Muddling Through,'" *Public Administration Review* 19(2) (1959): 79–88.

9 See https://en.wikiquote.org/w/index.php?title=H._L._Mencken&oldid=2093748.

10 K. M. Weick and K. M. Sutcliffe, *Managing the Unexpected: Assuring High Performance in an Age of Complexity* (San Francisco: Jossey-Bass, 2001).

11 S. Weiner and A. Schwartz, "Contextual Errors in Medical Decision Making: Overlooked and Understudied," *Academic Medicine: Journal of the Association of American Medical Colleges* 91(5) (2015).

12 This quote appears in the preface to W. James, *The Varieties of Religious Experience: A Study in Human Nature* (New York: W. W. Norton, 1902: repr., 1961).

13 I thank Kathryn Montgomery Hunter for this quote and the associated discussion in this paragraph from her blog exploring the nature of clinical practice, including decision making. See K. Montgomery, "Thinking about Thinking: Implications for Patient Safety," *Healthcare Quarterly* (Toronto, Canada) 12 (2008): e191–e194. The William James quote can be found in W. James, *William James: The Essential Writings* (Albany: State University of New York Press, 1986); W. M. James, "Brute and Human Intellect," *Journal of Speculative Philosophy* 12(3) (1878): 236–76; and W. James, "Brute and Human Intellect," in *William James: Writings, 1878–1899* (New York: Library of America, 1992), 11.

14 In that context, here are some other dilemmas that I faced in one day in the office. Do I suggest that a patient agree to take another round of potentially toxic chemotherapy knowing that it only has a 10 percent chance of helping? How frequent or "typical" does chest pain need to be to warrant an invasive procedure to determine whether serious heart disease is present? When do I prescribe narcotics for patients with intractable low-back pain, knowing that a small percentage of patients will become addicted? When do I assume that I should choose the treatment I used the last time I saw a patient similar to the current one, and when does that represent availability bias or some other form of self-deception?

15 Shared mind is when ideas, intuitions, and decisions emerge not only from individuals but from the interactions among them—an intersubjective experience.

R. M. Epstein and R. L. Street Jr., "Shared Mind: Communication, Decision Making, and Autonomy in Serious Illness," *Annals of Family Medicine* 9(5) (2011): 454–61; R. M. Epstein and R. E. Gramling, "What Is Shared in Shared Decision Making? Complex Decisions When the Evidence Is Unclear," *Medical Care Research and Review* 70(1S) (2012): 94–112; R. M. Epstein, "Whole Mind and Shared Mind in Clinical Decision-Making," *Patient Education & Counseling* 90(2) (2013): 200–206; and J. Zlatev et al., *The Shared Mind: Perspectives on Intersubjectivity* (Amsterdam and Philadelphia: John Benjamins, 2008.)

16 A provocative study using hyperscanning (two people in MRI scanners communicating with one another) showed that people whose brain activity is coordinated also are socially more connected. E. Bilek et al., "Information Flow between Interacting Human Brains: Identification, Validation, and Relationship to Social Expertise," *Proceedings of the National Academy of Sciences* 112(16) (2015): 5207–12.

17 L. R. Mujica-Parodi et al., "Chemosensory Cues to Conspecific Emotional Stress Activate Amygdala in Humans," *PLoS ONE* 4(7) (2009): e6415.

18 This vignette was adapted from F. Borrell-Carrió and R. M. Epstein, "Preventing Errors in Clinical Practice: A Call for Self-Awareness," *Annals of Family Medicine* 2(4) (2004): 310–16.

19 R. Srivastava, "Speaking Up—When Doctors Navigate Medical Hierarchy," *New England Journal of Medicine* 368(4) (2013): 302–5.

20 This quote, attributed to Dr. Faith Fitzgerald, appeared in A. K. Smith, D. B. White, and R. M. Arnold, "Uncertainty—the Other Side of Prognosis," *New England Journal of Medicine* 368(26) (2013): 2448–50.

21 F. Ismail-Beigi et al., "Individualizing Glycemic Targets in Type 2 Diabetes Mellitus: Implications of Recent Clinical Trials," *Annals of Internal Medicine* 154(8) (2011): 554–59.

22 D. L. Sackett et al., *Clinical Epidemiology: A Basic Science for Clinical Medicine*, 2nd ed. (Boston: Little, Brown, 1991).

23 G. Guyatt et al., "Patients at the Center: In Our Practice, and in Our Use of Language," *ACP Journal Club* 140(1) (2004): A11–A12. The presence of multiple conditions also affects patients' choices. See M. E. Tinetti, T. R. Fried, and C. M. Boyd, "Designing Health Care for the Most Common Chronic Condition—Multimorbidity," *JAMA* 307(23) (2012): 2493–94.

24 A. Tversky and D. Kahneman, "The Framing of Decisions and the Psychology of Choice," *Science* 211(4481) (1981): 453–58.

25 D. Kahneman, "A Perspective on Judgment and Choice: Mapping Bounded Rationality," *American Psychologist* 58(9) (2003): 697–720.

26 Croskerry suggests that enhancing metacognition would be a good thing for clinicians. If we could only understand our own biases during decision making, then we could have some hope of engaging in what Croskerry calls "de-biasing strategies" to make sounder and better-informed decisions by not only considering information and knowledge that we have, but how we select and use that knowledge and information. For Croskerry, who directs the Critical Thinking Program at Dalhousie University in Nova Scotia, de-biasing often involves switching from autopilot to "mindfulness of one's own thinking." See

P. Croskerry, "From Mindless to Mindful Practice—Cognitive Bias and Clinical Decision Making," *New England Journal of Medicine* 368(26) (2013): 2445–48.

27 Few interventions have shown promise in reducing implicit bias, and reduction in implicit bias has implications far beyond medicine. See Y. Kang, J. R. Gray, and J. F. Dovidio, "The Nondiscriminating Heart: Lovingkindness Meditation Training Decreases Implicit Intergroup Bias," *Journal of Experimental Psychology: General* 143(3) (2014): 1306; Y. Kang, J. Gruber, and J. R. Gray, "Mindfulness and De-automatization," *Emotion Review* 5(2) (2013): 192–201; A. Lueke and B. Gibson, "Mindfulness Meditation Reduces Implicit Age and Race Bias: The Role of Reduced Automaticity of Responding," *Social Psychology and Personality Science* (2014): 1–8; and A. C. Hafenbrack, Z. Kinias, and S. G. Barsade, "Debiasing the Mind through Meditation Mindfulness and the Sunk-Cost Bias," *Psychological Science* 25(2) (2014): 369–76.

28 G. Norman, M. Young, and L. Brooks, "Non-analytical Models of Clinical Reasoning: The Role of Experience," *Medical Education* 41(12) (2007): 1140–45.

29 See P. Croskerry, "A Universal Model of Diagnostic Reasoning," *Academic Medicine* 84(8) (2009): 1022–28.

30 J. M. Harlow, "Recovery after Severe Injury to the Head," *History of Psychiatry* (1993): 274–81 (originally published 1868 in the *Bulletin of the Massachusetts Medical Society*).

31 Epstein and Gramling, "What Is Shared in Shared Decision Making?"

32 S. Farber, "Living Every Minute," *Journal of Pain and Symptom Management* 49(4) (2015): 796–800.

33 K. Murray, "How Doctors Die—It's Not Like the Rest of Us, but It Should Be," *Zócalo Public Square*, November 30, 2011, 1775 77.

7. RESPONDING TO SUFFERING

1 The ideas in this chapter germinated with and expand on an article I coauthored with Tony Back, whom I acknowledge with gratitude, as part of a larger project on suffering and compassion in health care. See R. M. Epstein and A. L. Back, "Responding to Suffering," *JAMA* 314(24) (2015): 2623–24.

2 R. B. Haynes et al., "Increased Absenteeism from Work after Detection and Labeling of Hypertensive Patients," *New England Journal of Medicine* 299(14) (1978): 741–44; and J. E. Dimsdale, "Reflections on the Impact of Antihypertensive Medications on Mood, Sedation, and Neuropsychologic Functioning," *Archives of Internal Medicine* 152(1) (1992): 35–39.

3 A. W. Frank, "Can We Research Suffering?," *Qualitative Health Research* 11(3) (2001): 353–62.

4 E. J. Cassell, "The Nature of Suffering and the Goals of Medicine," *New England Journal of Medicine* 306(11) (1982): 639–45; E. J. Cassell, "Diagnosing Suffering: A Perspective," *Annals of Internal Medicine* 131(7) (1999): 531–34; and E. J. Cassell, "The Phenomenon of Suffering and Its Relationship to Pain," in *Handbook of Phenomenology and Medicine*, ed. S. K. Toombs (Dordrecht, Netherlands: Kluewer Academic Publishers, 2001), 371–90.

5 A slight misquote of Eldridge Cleaver, who said, "There is no more neutrality

in the world. You either have to be part of the solution, or you're going to be part of the problem." But he was not the first or the last to say this.

6 For further elaboration of this theme, see T. H. Lee, "The Word That Shall Not Be Spoken," *New England Journal of Medicine* 369(19) (2013): 1777–79.

7 There is a rich literature on the relationships among unexplained somatic symptoms, traumatic life events, mental illness, and functioning. See P. Salmon, "Patients Who Present Physical Symptoms in the Absence of Physical Pathology: A Challenge to Existing Models of Doctor-Patient Interaction," *Patient Education & Counseling* 39(1) (2000): 105–13; and W. Katon, M. Sullivan, and E. Walker, "Medical Symptoms without Identified Pathology: Relationship to Psychiatric Disorders, Childhood and Adult Trauma, and Personality Traits," *Annals of Internal Medicine* 134(9, pt. 2) (2001): 917–25. For a reference about how physicians respond to such patients, see E. A. Walker et al., "Predictors of Physician Frustration in the Care of Patients with Rheumatological Complaints," *General Hospital Psychiatry* 19(5) (1997): 315–23.

8 Clinicians reading this case report undoubtedly each have a theory of what else could have been done, an additional blood test or scan that would reveal the body's secrets and provide a clear path. Some may assert that the diagnosis is not recognized by mainstream medicine—due to an infectious agent, an environmental toxin, or a psychological process—nor is a humoral diagnosis according to traditional Chinese or ayurvedic medicine. Karen did explore many of these options. The point here is that the possibilities are endless, but investigating further always has a cost. Sometimes that cost is a side effect of a medication; other times it is in energy (seeing lots of doctors can be exhausting) or in finances or is existential (seeing oneself as diminished and fragmented rather than complete and whole).

9 Here are a few sources about the perils of labeling people "somatizers": R. M. Epstein, T. E. Quill, and I. R. McWhinney, "Somatization Reconsidered: Incorporating the Patient's Experience of Illness," *Archives of Internal Medicine* 159(3) (1999): 215–22; I. R. McWhinney, R. M. Epstein, and T. R. Freeman, "Rethinking Somatization," *Advances in Mind-Body Medicine* 17(4) (2001): 232–39; R. M. Epstein et al., "Physicians' Responses to Patients' Medically Unexplained Symptoms," *Psychosomatic Medicine* 68(2) (2006): 269–76; P. Salmon et al., "Doctors' Responses to Patients with Medically Unexplained Symptoms Who Seek Emotional Support: Criticism or Confrontation?," *General Hospital Psychiatry* 29(5) (2007): 454–60; and H. Waitzkin and H. Magana, "The Black Box in Somatization: Unexplained Physical Symptoms, Culture, and Narratives of Trauma," *Social Science & Medicine* 45(6) (1997): 811–25.

10 In her case, methotrexate, several TNF inhibitors, and a selective T-cell costimulation blocker.

11 I am grateful to Tony Back, who picked those words out when I was first recounting Karen's situation as part of an article we've coauthored for *JAMA*. See Epstein and Back, "Responding to Suffering."

12 Tony is also the founder of a new venture called VitalTalk, which offers training to physicians to help improve communication with patients during the most difficult moments.

13 A. L. Back et al., "'Why Are We Doing This?': Clinician Helplessness in the Face of Suffering," *Journal of Palliative Medicine* 18(1) (2015): 26–30.

14 S. E. Thorne et al., "'Being Known': Patients' Perspectives of the Dynamics of Human Connection in Cancer Care," *Psycho-Oncology* 14(10) (2005): 887–98.

15 Reference to Henry James noted in R. Charon, *Narrative Medicine: Honoring the Stories of Illness* (London: Oxford University Press, 2006).

16 J. Coulehan, "Compassionate Solidarity: Suffering, Poetry, and Medicine," *Perspectives in Biology and Medicine* 52(4) (2009): 585–603.

17 M. L. Johansen et al., "'I Deal with the Small Things': The Doctor-Patient Relationship and Professional Identity in GPs' Stories of Cancer Care," *Health* 16(6) (2012): 569–84.

18 A. L. Back et al., "Compassionate Silence in the Patient-Clinician Encounter: A Contemplative Approach," *Journal of Palliative Medicine* 12(12) (2009): 1113–17.

19 A. M. Kleinman, *The Illness Narratives: Suffering, Healing, and the Human Condition* (New York: Basic Books, 1988).

20 Kübler-Ross's five stages of dying—denial, anger, bargaining, depression, acceptance—are described in E. Kübler-Ross, S. Wessler, and L. V. Avioli, "On Death and Dying," *JAMA* 221(1972): 174–79.

21 From "Do Not Go Gentle into the Night," in *The Poems of Dylan Thomas* (New York: New Directions, 1938).

22 L. M. Candib, "Working with Suffering," *Patient Education & Counseling* 48(1) (2002): 43–50.

8. THE SHAKY STATE OF COMPASSION

1 G. L. Engel, "The Need for a New Medical Model: A Challenge for Biomedicine," *Science* 196(4286) (1977): 129–36.

2 G. L. Engel, "From Biomedical to Biopsychosocial: Being Scientific in the Human Domain," *Psychosomatics* 38(6) (1997): 521–28.

3 D. L. Berry et al., "Clinicians Communicating with Patients Experiencing Cancer Pain," *Cancer Investigation* 21(3) (2003): 374–81.

4 G. E. Pence, "Can Compassion Be Taught?," *Journal of Medical Ethics* 9(4) (1983): 189–91.

5 B. A. Lown, J. Rosen, and J. Marttila, "An Agenda for Improving Compassionate Care: A Survey Shows About Half of Patients Say Such Care Is Missing," *Health Affairs* 30(9) (2011): 1772–78.

6 The Milgram experiments were conducted in the early 1960s, shortly after the trial of Nazi war criminal Adolf Eichmann, with the intention of proving that most citizens were vulnerable to ethical compromise. See S. Milgram, "Behavioral Study of Obedience," *Journal of Abnormal Psychology* (1963): 67371–78.

7 It remains controversial whether long-term psychological harm was inflicted on some of the participants and whether the research protocol violated ethical norms at the time. Yet, this study prompted strict rules about informed consent for and the ethical review of all behavioral research.

8 J. M. Darley and C. D. Batson, "'From Jerusalem to Jericho': A Study of Situ-

ation and Dispositional Variables in Helping Behavior," *Journal of Personality and Social Psychology* 27(1) (1973): 100–108.

9 For one recent example, see A. Schattner, "My Most Informative Error," *JAMA Internal Medicine* 175(5) (2015): 681.

10 J. Halifax, "A Heuristic Model of Enactive Compassion," *Current Opinion in Supportive and Palliative Care* 6(2) (2012): 228–35. Also, see her book *Being with Dying* (Boulder, CO: Shambhala Publications, 2008). For an understanding of how one can empathize with someone whom we perceive as different, see C. Lamm, A. N. Meltzoff, and J. Decety, "How Do We Empathize with Someone Who Is Not Like Us? A Functional Magnetic Resonance Imaging Study," *Journal of Cognitive Neuroscience* 22(2) (2010): 362–76.

11 H. Fukushima, Y. Terasawa, and S. Umeda, "Association between Interoception and Empathy: Evidence from Heartbeat-Evoked Brain Potential," *International Journal of Psychophysiology* 79(2) (2011): 259–65; and T. Singer, H. D. Critchley, and K. Preuschoff, "A Common Role of Insula in Feelings, Empathy and Uncertainty," *Trends in Cognitive Sciences* 13(8) (2009): 334–40.

12 C. Lamm, C. D. Batson, and J. Decety, "The Neural Substrate of Human Empathy: Effects of Perspective-Taking and Cognitive Appraisal," *Journal of Cognitive Neuroscience* 19(1) (2007): 42–58.

13 H. De Jaegher and E. Di Paolo, "Participatory Sense-Making: An Enactive Approach to Social Cognition," *Phenomenology and the Cognitive Sciences* 6(4) (2007): 485–507.

14 For some illustrative examples of physician self-disclosure gone awry, see S. H. McDaniel et al., "'Enough about Me, Let's Get Back to You': Physician Self-Disclosure during Primary Care Encounters," *Annals of Internal Medicine* 149(11) (2008): 835–37.

15 A concise summary of these pathways linking the ventral striatum and the medial orbitofrontal cortex can be found in O. M. Klimecki et al., "Differential Pattern of Functional Brain Plasticity after Compassion and Empathy Training," *Social Cognitive and Affective Neuroscience* 9(6) (2014): 873–79.

16 See M. Hojat et al., "The Devil Is in the Third Year: A Longitudinal Study of Erosion of Empathy in Medical School," *Academic Medicine* 84(9) (2009): 1182–91.

17 D. C. Batson, "These Things Called Empathy: Eight Related but Distinct Phenomena," in *The Social Neuroscience of Empathy*, eds. J. Decety and W. Ickes (Denver, CO: Bradford, 2009), chap. 1, 13–15; Lamm, Batson, and Decety, "Neural Substrate of Human Empathy"; and N. Eisenberg and N. D. Eggum, "Empathic Responding: Sympathy and Personal Distress," in *Social Neuroscience of Empathy*, eds. Decety and Ickes, chap. 6, 71–83.

18 For recommendations on how clinicians can use self-disclosure more effectively, see McDaniel et al., "'Enough about Me.'"

19 J. Halpern, "What Is Clinical Empathy?," *Journal of General Internal Medicine* 18(8) (2003): 670–74.

20 M. K. Kearney et al., "Self-Care of Physicians Caring for Patients at the End of Life: 'Being Connected . . . a Key to My Survival,'" *JAMA* 301(11) (2009): 1155–64.

21 J. Decety and C. Lamm, "Empathy versus Personal Distress: Recent Evidence from Social Neuroscience," in *Social Neuroscience of Empathy*, eds. Decety and Ickes, chap. 15, 199–213.

22 S. Salzberg, *Lovingkindness: The Revolutionary Art of Happiness* (Boston: Shambhala, 1997).

23 These areas would be the anterior insula and anterior midcingulate cortex.

24 The dopamine, opioid, and oxytocin centers.

25 F. de Vignemont and T. Singer, "The Empathic Brain: How, When and Why?," *Trends in Cognitive Sciences* 10(10) (2006): 435–41.

26 Salzberg, *Lovingkindness.*

27 Aristotle, *The Nicomachean Ethics,* trans. David Ross, revised with an introduction and notes by Lesley Brown (New York: Oxford University Press, 2009); and T. J. Oord, *Defining Love: A Philosophical, Scientific, and Theological Engagement* (Grand Rapids, MI: Brazos Press, 2010).

28 Here, the work of psychologist Tania Singer at the Max Planck Institute in Leipzig, Germany, is particularly relevant. Singer reported results of an experiment in which people who had never done any kind of meditation agreed to participate in a nine-month program. For three months they practiced focused attention training, alone at home and in group sessions. Then for another three months they practiced a form of dyadic attention training—"attentive listening" to others through structured dialogues conducted in person or by phone. For the final three months they engaged in traditional compassion practice. Singer and her team found that the effects of each contemplative practice built a particular set of skills. Focused attention training enhanced attentional networks and reduced distractibility. Compassion practice had greater effects on pro-social attitudes such as caring and concern for others and desire to ameliorate others' suffering. Singer's study was done with ordinary people from a variety of walks of life, yet could easily apply to those who work in medical settings. See T. Singer and M. Bolz, *Compassion: Bridging Practice and Science* (Munich, Germany: Max Planck Society, 2013).

29 For further information, see H. G. Engen and T. Singer, "Compassion-Based Emotion Regulation Up-Regulates Experienced Positive Affect and Associated Neural Networks," *Social Cognitive and Affective Neuroscience* 10(9) (2015): 1291–301.

30 H. Y. Weng et al., "Compassion Training Alters Altruism and Neural Responses to Suffering," *Psychological Science* 24(7) (2013): 1171–80.

9. WHEN BAD THINGS HAPPEN

1 L. T. Kohn, J. M. Corrigan, and M. S. Donaldson, *To Err Is Human: Building a Safer Health System* (Washington, DC: National Academy Press, 2000).

2 T. H. Gallagher et al., "Patients' and Physicians' Attitudes regarding the Disclosure of Medical Errors," *JAMA* 289(8) (2003): 1001–7.

3 Kohn, Corrigan, and Donaldson, *To Err Is Human.*

4 In this chapter most of the examples about errors that I have chosen are ambiguous. This was intentional. Dramatic errors due to gross incompetence or

neglect—such as amputating the wrong leg or giving a lethal dose of a medication—are uncommon, and the brute force of the litigation system can override mindful attempts to restore balance and connection. In fact, though, much of the total burden to patients and clinicians from bad outcomes results from a combination of small lapses in attention, unfortunate coincidences, miscommunicated intentions, and team and systems failures.

5 H. B. Beckman et al., "The Doctor-Patient Relationship and Malpractice: Lessons from Plaintiff Depositions," *Archives of Internal Medicine* 154(12) (1994): 1365–70.

6 B. Ho and E. Liu, "Does Sorry Work? The Impact of Apology Laws on Medical Malpractice," *Journal of Risk and Uncertainty* 43(2) (2011): 141–67.

7 N. M. Saitta and S. D. Hodge, "Is It Unrealistic to Expect a Doctor to Apologize for an Unforeseen Medical Complication?—a Primer on Apologies Laws," *Pennsylvania Bar Association Quarterly* (2011): 93–110.

8 N. M. Saitta and S. Hodge, "Physician Apologies," *Practical Lawyer*, December 2011, 35–43; and N. Saitta and S. D. Hodge, "Efficacy of a Physician's Words of Empathy: An Overview of State Apology Laws," *Journal of the American Osteopathic Association* 112(5) (2012): 302–6.

9 A. D. Waterman et al., "The Emotional Impact of Medical Errors on Practicing Physicians in the United States and Canada," *Joint Commission Journal on Quality and Patient Safety* 33(8) (2007): 467–76.

10 A. W. Wu, "Medical Error: The Second Victim. The Doctor Who Makes the Mistake Needs Help Too," *Western Journal of Medicine* 172(6) (2000): 358.

11 M. P. Stiegler, "A Piece of My Mind. What I Learned about Adverse Events from Captain Sully: It's Not What You Think," *JAMA* 313(4) (2015): 361–62.

12 S. K. Howard et al., "Anesthesia Crisis Resource Management Training: Teaching Anesthesiologists to Handle Critical Incidents," *Aviation, Space, and Environmental Medicine* 63(9) (1992): 763–70.

13 C. P. West et al., "Association of Perceived Medical Errors with Resident Distress and Empathy: A Prospective Longitudinal Study," *JAMA* 296(9) (2006): 1071–78.

14 In her thoughtful article about the program, Karan reported that a resident drew up medications into two syringes then forgot to mark which drug was in which syringe; another resident administered an entire syringe of a powerful stimulant thinking it was saline solution; another noted that blood-pressure cuffs in the operating room had "questionable" stains on them, likely another patient's blood; and so forth. See S. B. Karan, J. S. Berger, and M. Wajda, "Confessions of Physicians: What Systemic Reporting Does Not Uncover," *Journal of Graduate Medical Education* 7(4) (2015): 528–30.

15 L. Granek, "When Doctors Grieve," *New York Times*, May 27, 2012; and L. Granek et al., "Nature and Impact of Grief over Patient Loss on Oncologists' Personal and Professional Lives," *Archives of Internal Medicine* 172(12) (2012): 964–66.

16 R. A. Rodenbach et al., "Relationships between Personal Attitudes about Death and Communication with Terminally Ill Patients: How Oncology Clinicians Grapple with Mortality," *Patient Education & Counseling* 99(3) (2015): 356–63.

17 L. Granek et al., "What Do Oncologists Want?," *Supportive Care in Cancer* 20(10) (2012): 2627–32.

18 M. Shayne and T. E. Quill, "Oncologists Responding to Grief," *Archives of Internal Medicine* 172(12) (2012): 966–67.

19 C. K. Germer, *The Mindful Path to Self-Compassion: Freeing Yourself from Destructive Thoughts and Emotions* (New York: Guilford Press, 2009); and K. D. Neff and C. K. Germer, "A Pilot Study and Randomized Controlled Trial of the Mindful Self-Compassion Program," *Journal of Clinical Pscyhology* 69(1) (2013): 28–44.

20 K. D. Neff, Y.-P. Hsieh, and K. Dejitterat, "Self-Compassion, Achievement Goals, and Coping with Academic Failure," *Self and Identity* 4(3) (2005): 263–87; Neff and Germer, "Pilot Study and Randomized Controlled Trial"; and M. R. Leary et al., "Self-Compassion and Reactions to Unpleasant Self-Relevant Events: The Implications of Treating Oneself Kindly," *Journal of Personality and Social Psychology* 92(5) (2007): 887.

21 M. Lesser, *Know Yourself, Forget Yourself: Five Truths to Transform Your Work, Relationships, and Everyday Life* (Novato, CA: New World Library, 2013).

22 S. D. Scott et al., "The Natural History of Recovery for the Healthcare Provider 'Second Victim' after Adverse Patient Events," *Quality and Safety in Health Care* 18(5) (2009): 325–30.

23 See http://www.brighamandwomens.org/medical_professionals/career/cpps /default.aspx.

24 The San Francisco Department of Public Health has developed a Trauma Informed Systems (TIS) framework, intended to help improve organizational functioning, increase resilience, and improve workforce experience. This includes mandatory foundational training to all nine thousand public health employees to create a shared language and understanding of trauma, a Champions Learning Community (CLC), a train-the-trainer program, intentional efforts to align TIS with all workforce and policy initiatives, and leadership engagement and outreach to support integration of TIS principles into day-to-day operations as well as promote system change at the program and policy level.

10. HEALING THE HEALER

1 This was quoted in *JAMA* 189 (1964): 97.

2 To give just one of many examples, care for patients with diabetes in primary care is typically measured according to the frequency of testing for hemoglobin A1c, a marker for long-term control of diabetes. Some clinics actually use the test results (normal vs. high vs. very high) as the quality metric. However, frequency of testing does not reliably predict control of diabetes, and long-term outcomes for many people over age sixty-five with type 2 diabetes is minimally affected by whether the A1c level is below 7 (considered optimal) or if it's closer to 8 (considered poor care), and in some cases higher levels are desirable if there is risk of *low* blood sugar. The factors that go into control

of blood sugar go well beyond the prescription pad and are usually unreimbursed (e.g., exercise programs, nutritional counseling, social support). Conversely, the quality of physician empathy is a powerful factor in blood sugar control in patients with diabetes, yet goes unmeasured and unreimbursed. See M. Hojat et al., "Physicians' Empathy and Clinical Outcomes for Diabetic Patients," *Academic Medicine* 86(3) (2011): 359–64.

3 Moral distress—when people are put in situations in which they're kept from doing what they know is right or are forced to do things that conflict with their values—can be blatant, such as being told to deny a patient needed pain medication, or more insidious. See A. Catlin et al., "Conscientious Objection: A Potential Neonatal Nursing Response to Care Orders That Cause Suffering at the End of Life? Study of a Concept," *Neonatal Network—Journal of Neonatal Nursing* 27(2) (2008): 101–8; L. H. Pololi et al., "Why Are a Quarter of Faculty Considering Leaving Academic Medicine? A Study of Their Perceptions of Institutional Culture and Intentions to Leave at 26 Representative US Medical Schools," *Academic Medicine* 87(7) (2012): 859–69; C. H. Rushton, A. W. Kaszniak, and J. S. Halifax, "Addressing Moral Distress: Application of a Framework to Palliative Care Practice," *Journal of Palliative Medicine* 16(9) (2013): 1080–88; C. H. Rushton, A. W. Kaszniak, and J. S. Halifax, "A Framework for Understanding Moral Distress among Palliative Care Clinicians," *Journal of Palliative Medicine* 16(9) (2013): 1074–79; and C. Varcoe et al., "Nurses' Perceptions of and Responses to Morally Distressing Situations," *Nursing Ethics* 19(4) (2012): 488–500.

4 Burnout gets worse toward midcareer, as clinical and administrative responsibilities increase while other aspects of life become more complex. Some surveys suggest that women are more burned out than men, which is understandable given their more complex social roles and responsibilities—and other surveys suggest that they are also more resilient. See T. D. Shanafelt et al., "Changes in Burnout and Satisfaction with Work-Life Balance in Physicians and the General US Working Population between 2011 and 2014," *Mayo Clinic Proceedings* 90(12) (2015): 1600–1613; and http://www.medscape.com /features/slideshow/lifestyle/2016/public/overview#page=1 for 2016 statistics on physician burnout, overall and by physician specialty. Also see M. W. C. Friedberg, PG, K. R. VanBusum, F. M. Aunon, C. Pham, J. P. Caloyeras, S. Mattke, E. Pitchforth, D. D. Quigley, and R. H. Brook, "Factors Affecting Physician Professional Satisfaction and Their Implications for Patient Care, Health Systems, and Health Policy," 2013, http://www.rand.org/con tent/dam/rand/pubs/research_reports/RR400/RR439/RAND_RR439.pdf; "Physician Wellness Services and Cejka Search: 2011 Physician Stress and Burnout Survey," 2011, http://www.cejkasearch.com/wp-content/uploads /physician-stress-burnout-survey.pdf; and Physicians Foundation, "A Survey of America's Physicians: Practice Patterns and Perspectives, an Examination of the Professional Morale, Practice Patterns, Career Plans, and Healthcare Perspectives of Today's Physicians, Aggregated by Age, Gender, Primary Care /Specialists, and Practice Owners/Employees," 2012, http://www.physicians foundation.org/uploads/default/Physicians_Foundation_2012_Biennial _Survey.pdf. An article in the November 2014 *Atlantic* cites five current books

in the popular press documenting the devastating consequences of physician burnout. See M. O'Rourke, "Doctors Tell All—and It's Bad," *Atlantic*, November 2014, http://www.theatlantic.com/magazine/archive/2014/11/doctors-tell-all-and-its-bad/380785/; and D. Ofri, "The Epidemic of Disillusioned Doctors," *Time*, published electronically July 2, 2013, http://ideas.time.com/2013/07/02/the-epidemic-of-disillusioned-doctors.

5 M. D. McHugh et al., "Nurses' Widespread Job Dissatisfaction, Burnout, and Frustration with Health Benefits Signal Problems for Patient Care," *Health Affairs* 30(2) (2011): 202–10; and C. A. J. Dixon et al., "Abusive Behaviour Experienced by Primary Care Receptionists: A Cross-Sectional Survey," *Family Practice* 21(2) (2004): 137–39.

6 Most of the work on physician burnout has been done by a research group at the Mayo Clinic in Minnesota and the Physicians Worklife Study, with some important studies done by other groups. See L. N. Dyrbye et al., "Relationship between Burnout and Professional Conduct and Attitudes among US Medical Students," *JAMA* 304(11) (2010): 1173–80; L. N. Dyrbye et al., "Burnout and Suicidal Ideation among US Medical Students," *Annals of Internal Medicine* 149(5) (2008): 334–41; L. N. Dyrbye et al., "Physician Satisfaction and Burnout at Different Career Stages," *Mayo Clinic Proceedings* 88(12) (2013): 1358–67; A. M. Fahrenkopf et al., "Rates of Medication Errors among Depressed and Burnt Out Residents: Prospective Cohort Study," *BMJ* 1(7642) (2008): 488–91; S. Gabel, "Demoralization: A Precursor to Physician Burnout?," *American Family Physician* 86(9) (2012): 861–62; L. N. Dyrbye et al., "Burnout among US Medical Students, Residents, and Early Career Physicians Relative to the General US Population," *Academic Medicine* 89(3) (2014): 443–51; T. D. Shanafelt et al., "Career Fit and Burnout among Academic Faculty," *Archives of Internal Medicine* 169(10) (2009): 990–95; C. P. West et al., "Association of Resident Fatigue and Distress with Perceived Medical Errors," *JAMA* 302(12) (2009): 1294–300; M. Linzer et al., "Predicting and Preventing Physician Burnout: Results from the United States and the Netherlands," *American Journal of Medicine* 111(2) (2001): 170–75; J. E. McMurray et al., "The Work Lives of Women Physicians: Results from the Physician Work Life Study. The SGIM Career Satisfaction Study Group," *Journal of General Internal Medicine* 15(6) (2000): 372–80; E. Williams et al., "The Relationship of Organizational Culture, Stress, Satisfaction, and Burnout with Physician-Reported Error and Suboptimal Patient Care: Results from the Memo Study," *Health Care Management Review* 32(3) (2007): 203–12; and E. S. Williams et al., "Understanding Physicians' Intentions to Withdraw from Practice: The Role of Job Satisfaction, Job Stress, Mental and Physical Health," *Health Care Management Review* 26(1) (2001): 7–19.

7 T. Kushnir et al., "Is Burnout Associated with Referral Rates among Primary Care Physicians in Community Clinics?," *Family Practice* 31(1) (2014): 44–50; K. H. Bachman and D. K. Freeborn, "HMO Physicians' Use of Referrals," *Social Science & Medicine* 48(4) (1999): 547–57; and B. E. Sirovich, S. Woloshin, and L. M. Schwartz, "Too Little? Too Much? Primary Care Physicians' Views on US Health Care: A Brief Report," *Archives of Internal Medicine* 171(17) (2011): 1582–85.

8 See J. S. Haas et al., "Is the Professional Satisfaction of General Internists Associated with Patient Satisfaction?," *Journal of General Internal Medicine* 15(2) (2000): 122–28.

9 Most of these will continue to practice medicine but not primary care. Many choose urgent care and hospital medicine. Some take on administrative roles.

10 R. L. Lichtenstein, "Review Article: The Job Satisfaction and Retention of Physicians in Organized Settings: A Literature Review," *Medical Care Research and Review* 41(3) (1984): 139–79; J. E. Berger and R. L. Boyle Jr., "How to Avoid the High Costs of Physician Turnover," *Medical Group Management Journal* 39(6) (1991): 80–82; S. B. Buchbinder et al., "Estimates of Costs of Primary Care Physician Turnover," *American Journal of Managed Care* 5(11) (1999): 1431–38; and J. D. Waldman et al., "The Shocking Cost of Turnover in Health Care," *Health Care Management Review* 29(1) (2004): 2–7.

11 R. G. Hill Jr., L. M. Sears, and S. W. Melanson, "4,000 Clicks: A Productivity Analysis of Electronic Medical Records in a Community Hospital ED," *American Journal of Emergency Medicine* 31(11) (2013): 1591–94; and S. Babbott et al., "Electronic Medical Records and Physician Stress in Primary Care: Results from the Memo Study," *Journal of the American Medical Informatics Association* 21(e1) (2014): e100–e106.

12 C. Maslach, "Job Burnout," *Current Directions in Psychological Science* 12(5) (2003): 189–92.

13 A. Spickard Jr., S. G. Gabbe, and J. F. Christensen, "Mid-Career Burnout in Generalist and Specialist Physicians," *JAMA* 288(12) (2002): 1447–50.

14 Dyrbye et al., "Burnout and Suicidal Ideation."

15 L. Y. Abramson, M. E. Seligman, and J. D. Teasdale, "Learned Helplessness in Humans: Critique and Reformulation," *Journal of Abnormal Psychology* 87(1) (1978): 49–74.

16 For a discussion of physicians' psychological vulnerabilities, see A. Nedrow, N. A. Steckler, and J. Hardman, "Physician Resilience and Burnout: Can You Make the Switch?," *Family Practice Management* 20(1) (2013): 25–30; and G. E. Vaillant, N. C. Sobowale, and C. McArthur, "Some Psychologic Vulnerabilities of Physicians," *New England Journal of Medicine* 287 (1972): 372–75.

17 Physicians' overtesting is not entirely driven by fear of malpractice lawsuits. This behavior is also common among doctors in countries with low rates of malpractice litigation. See G. O. Gabbard, "The Role of Compulsiveness in the Normal Physician," *JAMA* 254(20) (1985): 2926–29.

18 See J. Legassie, E. M. Zibrowski, and M. A. Goldszmidt, "Measuring Resident Well-Being: Impostorism and Burnout Syndrome in Residency," *Journal of General Internal Medicine* 23(7) (2008): 1090–94; and P. R. Clance, *The Impostor Phenomenon: When Success Makes You Feel Like a Fake* (New York: Bantam Books, 1986).

19 For further discussion, see A. D. Mancini and G. A. Bonanno, "Predictors and Parameters of Resilience to Loss: Toward an Individual Differences Model," *Journal of Personality* 77(6) (2009): 1805–32.

20 J. Halifax, "A Heuristic Model of Enactive Compassion," *Current Opinion in Supportive and Palliative Care* 6(2) (2012): 228–35.

21 See the "A Piece of My Mind" sections of *JAMA* and "On Being a Doctor" sections of the *Annals of Internal Medicine*.

22 N. N. Taleb, *Antifragile: Things That Gain from Disorder* (New York: Random House, 2014).

23 S. M. Southwick and D. S. Charney, *Resilience: The Science of Mastering Life's Greatest Challenges* (Cambridge: Cambridge University Press, 2012).

24 S. J. Russo et al., "Neurobiology of Resilience," *Nature Neuroscience* 15(11) (2012): 1475–84.

25 Self-determination theory, a psychological model developed at the University of Rochester, suggests that a sense of autonomy (rather than a sense of feeling controlled), a sense that you're competent and have the skills to reach your goals, and strong caring relationships with others would be associated with greater resilience. See E. L. Deci and R. M. Ryan, *Intrinsic Motivation and Self-Determination in Human Behavior* (New York: Plenum Press, 1985).

26 D. Cicchetti and F. A. Rogosch, "Gene × Environment Interaction and Resilience: Effects of Child Maltreatment and Serotonin, Corticotropin Releasing Hormone, Dopamine, and Oxytocin Genes," *Development and Psychopathology* 24(02) (2012): 411–27; A. Feder, E. J. Nestler, and D. S. Charney, "Psychobiology and Molecular Genetics of Resilience," *Nature Reviews Neuroscience* 10(6) (2009): 446–57; and Russo et al., "Neurobiology of Resilience."

27 D. C. Johnson et al., "Modifying Resilience Mechanisms in At-Risk Individuals: A Controlled Study of Mindfulness Training in Marines Preparing for Deployment," *American Journal of Psychiatry* 171(8) (2014): 844–53; G. Wu et al., "Understanding Resilience," *Frontiers in Behavioral Neuroscience* 7(10) (2013); and Russo et al., "Neurobiology of Resilience."

28 K. Olson, K. J. Kemper, and J. D. Mahan, "What Factors Promote Resilience and Protect against Burnout in First-Year Pediatric and Medicine-Pediatric Residents?," *Journal of Evidence-Based Complementary and Alternative Medicine* 20(3) (2015): 192–98; K. J. Kemper and M. Khirallah, "Acute Effects of Online Mind-Body Skills Training on Resilience, Mindfulness, and Empathy," *Journal of Evidence-Based Complementary and Alternative Medicine* 20(4) (2015): 247–53; J. T. Thomas, "Intrapsychic Predictors of Professional Quality of Life: Mindfulness, Empathy, and Emotional Separation" (Lexington: University of Kentucky, 2011); and Johnson et al., "Modifying Resilience Mechanisms."

29 H. B. Beckman et al., "The Impact of a Program in Mindful Communciation on Primary Care Physicians," *Academic Medicine* 87(6) (2012): 1–5; and M. S. Krasner et al., "Association of an Educational Program in Mindful Communication with Burnout, Empathy, and Attitudes among Primary Care Physicians," *JAMA* 302(12) (2009): 1284–93. The Big Five personality factors are neuroticism, extraversion, openness to experience, agreeableness, and conscientiousness. Focused attention is one facet of conscientiousness and mental stability is one facet of (lack of) neuroticism.

30 A. Caspi and B. W. Roberts, "Personality Development across the Life Course: The Argument for Change and Continuity," *Psychological Inquiry* 12(2) (2001): 49–66.

31 The opposite—workaholics who get fulfillment only at work and see home life as dull—are equally deprived of the richness that life can offer.

32 See http://www.marclesser.net/tag/work-life-balance. I mentioned Marc Lesser in chapter 9. Marc is a Zen priest who runs mindfulness programs for Fortune 500 companies.

33 K. W. Brown and R. M. Ryan, "The Benefits of Being Present: Mindfulness and Its Role in Psychological Well-Being," *Journal of Personality and Social Psychology* 84(4) (2003): 822–48; and N. Weinstein and R. M. Ryan, "When Helping Helps: Autonomous Motivation for Prosocial Behavior and Its Influence on Well-Being for the Helper and Recipient," *Journal of Personality and Social Psychology* 98(2) (2010): 222–44.

34 Shanafelt et al., "Career Fit and Burnout."

35 For a copy, see C. Maslach, S. Jackson, and M. Leiter, "Maslach Burnout Inventory: Third Edition," in *Evaluating Stress: A Book of Resources*, eds. C. P. Zalaquett and R. J. Wood (Lanham, MD: Scarecrow Press, 1998), 191–218; and C. Maslach, W. B. Schaufeli, and M. P. Leiter, "Job Burnout," *Annual Review of Psychology* (2001): 52397–422.

36 Our understanding of what these structures do and how they interact is still rudimentary, and we are a long way from knowing, for example, whether the activation of some of these structures is the cause or the effect of particular mental states. And, while neuroimaging is merely a *marker* for changes in the brain—you cannot actually "see" a thought or an emotion—the results of these experiments are nonetheless compelling. See B. K. Hölzel et al., "How Does Mindfulness Meditation Work? Proposing Mechanisms of Action from a Conceptual and Neural Perspective," *Perspectives on Psychological Science* 6(6) (2011): 537–59; D. Vago and D. Silbersweig, "Self-Awareness, Self-Regulation, and Self-Transcendence (S-Art): A Framework for Understanding the Neurobiological Mechanisms of Mindfulness," *Frontiers in Human Neuroscience* 6(296) (2012): 1–6; and R. J. Davidson et al., "Alterations in Brain and Immune Function Produced by Mindfulness Meditation," *Psychosomatic Medicine* 65(4) (2003): 564–70; Y.-Y. Tang, B. K. Hölzel, and M. I. Posner, "The Neuroscience of Mindfulness Meditation," *Nature Reviews Neuroscience* 16(4) (2015): 213–25; and A. Brewer and K. Garrison, "The Posterior Cingulate Cortex as a Plausible Mechanistic Target of Meditation: Findings from Neuroimaging," *Annals of the New York Academy of Sciences* 1307(1) (2014): 19–27.

37 See D. C. Johnson et al., "Modifying Resilience Mechanisms"; E. A. Stanley et al., "Mindfulness-Based Mind Fitness Training: A Case Study of a High Stress Pre-deployment Military Cohort," *Cognitive and Behavioral Practice* 18(4) (2011): 566–76; E. A. Stanley, "Mindfulness-Based Mind Fitness Training (MMFT): An Approach for Enhancing Performance and Building Resilience in High Stress Contexts," in *The Wiley Blackwell Handbook of Mindfulness*, eds. A. Ie, C. T. Ngnoumen, and E. J. Langer (Hoboken, NJ: Wiley, 2014), 964–85; A. P. Jha et al., "Examining the Protective Effects of Mindfulness Training on Working Memory Capacity and Affective Experience," *Emotion* 10(1) (2010): 54–64; and A. P. Jha et al., "Minds 'at Attention': Mindfulness Training Curbs Attentional Lapses in Military Cohorts," *PLoS ONE* 10(2) (2015): e0116889.

11. BECOMING MINDFUL

1 E. A. Maguire, K. Woollett, and H. J. Spiers, "London Taxi Drivers and Bus Drivers: A Structural MRI and Neuropsychological Analysis," *Hippocampus* 16(12) (2006): 1091–101.

2 K. Woollett and E. A. Maguire, "Acquiring 'the Knowledge' of London's Layout Drives Structural Brain Changes," *Current Biology* 21(24) (2011): 2109–14.

3 This famous postulate of neuroscience is attributed to Carla Shatz at Stanford University (see C. J. Shatz, "The Developing Brain," *Scientific American* 267(3) (1992): 60–67) and is based on a theory of learning proposed by Donald Hebb in 1949. See D. Hebb, *The Organization of Behavior* (New York: Wiley, 1949). "Wiring together" is positive when it promotes acquisition of skills or habits of mind, but problematic when "firing together" reinforces unwanted mental rumination, obsessions, compulsions, anxiety, and depression.

4 K. A. Ericsson, "An Expert-Performance Perspective of Research on Medical Expertise: The Study of Clinical Performance," *Medical Education* 41(12) (2007): 1124–30. Much of the argument in the next few paragraphs is summarized in A. S. O. Leung, C. A. Moulton, and R. M. Epstein, "The Competent Mind: Beyond Cognition," in *The Question of Competence: Reconsidering Medical Education in the Twenty-First Century*, eds. B. D. Hodges and L. Lingard (Ithaca and London: Cornell University Press, 2012), chap. 7, 155–76.

5 G. L. Engel, "What If Music Students Were Taught to Play Their Instruments as Medical Students Are Taught to Interview?," *Pharos of Alpha Omega Alpha Honor Medical Society* (1982): 4512–13.

6 H. L. Dreyfus, *On the Internet (Thinking in Action)* (New York: Routledge, 2001).

7 See Leung, Moulton, and Epstein, "Competent Mind."

8 For a discussion of adaptive expertise, see G. Hatano and K. Inagaki, "Child Development and Education in Japan," in *Two Courses of Expertise*, eds. H. Stevenson, H. Azuma, and K. Hakuta (New York: Freeman, 1986), 262–72. For a richer discussion of context, see S. Weiner and A. Schwartz, "Contextual Errors in Medical Decision Making: Overlooked and Understudied," *Academic Medicine: Journal of the Association of American Medical Colleges* 91(5) (2016): 657–62.

9 The parallels between jazz and clinical practice have been described in two wonderful articles listed below. Importantly, the ability to improvise depends on years of practice and assimilating the rules of harmony and structure of the music. See P. Haidet, "Jazz and the 'Art' of Medicine: Improvisation in the Medical Encounter," *Annals of Family Medicine* 5(2) (2007): 164–69; and A. F. Shaughnessy, D. C. Slawson, and L. Becker, "Clinical Jazz: Harmonizing Clinical Experience and Evidence-Based Medicine," *Journal of Family Practice* 47(6) (1998): 425–28.

10 W. James, *The Principles of Psychology* (Cambridge, MA: Harvard University Press, 1981).

11 Y.-Y. Tang et al., "Short-Term Meditation Training Improves Attention and Self-Regulation," *Proceedings of the National Academy of Sciences* 104(43) (2007): 17152–56; and Y.-Y. Tang et al., "Central and Autonomic Nervous

System Interaction Is Altered by Short-Term Meditation," *Proceedings of the National Academy of Sciences* 106(22) (2009): 8865–70.

12 D. M. Levy et al., "The Effects of Mindfulness Meditation Training on Multitasking in a High-Stress Information Environment," in *Proceedings of Graphics Interface 2012* (Toronto: Canadian Information Processing Society, 2012), 45–52; R. J. Davidson and A. W. Kaserniak, "Conceptual and Methodological Issues in Research on Mindfulness and Meditation," *American Psychologist* 70(7) (2015): 581–92; B. K. Hölzel et al., "How Does Mindfulness Meditation Work? Proposing Mechanisms of Action from a Conceptual and Neural Perspective," *Perspectives on Psychological Science* 6(6) (2011): 537–59; and Y.-Y. Tang, B. K. Hölzel, and M. I. Posner, "The Neuroscience of Mindfulness Meditation," *Nature Reviews Neuroscience* 16(4) (2015): 213–25.

13 A description of ten stages of attention training, practices used to achieve them, and their implications for living one's life can be found in B. A. Wallace, *The Attention Revolution: Unlocking the Power of the Focused Mind* (Somerville, MA: Wisdom Publications, 2006). The ten stages of attention are directed, continuous, resurgent, close, tamed, pacified, fully pacified, and single-pointed attention, then attentional balance and "shamatha."

14 A. W. Kaserniak, "Meditation, Mindfulness, Cognition, and Emotion: Implications for Community-Based Older Adult Programs," in *Enhancing Cognitive Fitness in Adults*, eds. P. E. Hartman-Stein and A. LaRue (New York: Springer, 2011), chap. 5, 85–104.

15 The word *mindfulness* also can be confusing. People commonly use it to describe a relatively fixed personality trait, a state of mind that can be achieved, and also a specific set of practices such as meditation. Any number of everyday activities can become mindful practices—one can play tennis mindfully, run mindfully, cook and eat mindfully, read poetry mindfully, and listen to or make music mindfully. I prefer what is now considered to be the original meaning of the Pali word *sati*—"remembering"—remembering who you are and what is important, every moment of every day.

16 Jon Kabat-Zinn is responsible for having secularized meditation traditions that originated in South and Southeast Asia and made them accessible to the general Western public. See J. Kabat-Zinn, *Full Catastrophe Living: Using the Wisdom of Your Body and Mind to Face Stress, Pain, and Illness* (New York: Bantam Dell, 1990).

17 For two explorations of how one can engage in awareness practice without adhering to an organized belief system, see S. Batchelor, *Buddhism without Beliefs: A Contemporary Guide to Awakening* (New York: Riverhead Books, 1997); and S. Harris, *Waking Up: A Guide to Spirituality without Religion* (New York: Simon & Schuster, 2015).

18 These pathways are not as well elaborated as attentional pathways and represent a cutting edge of neuroscience research. O. M. Klimecki et al., "Differential Pattern of Functional Brain Plasticity after Compassion and Empathy Training," *Social Cognitive and Affective Neuroscience* 9(6) (2014): 873–79.

19 D. A. Schroeder et al., "A Brief Mindfulness-Based Intervention for Primary Care Physicians: A Pilot Randomized Controlled Trial," *American Journal of Lifestyle Medicine* (2016): 1–9.

20 S. B. Goldberg et al., "The Secret Ingredient in Mindfulness Interventions? A Case for Practice Quality over Quantity," *Journal of Counseling Psychology* 61(3) (2014): 491–97.

21 For very readable introductions into this complex realm, see A. R. Damasio, *Descartes' Error: Emotion, Reason, and the Human Brain* (New York: G. P. Putnam's Sons, 1994); and A. R. Damasio, *The Feeling of What Happens: Body and Emotion in the Making of Consciousness* (New York: Harcourt Brace, 1999). While some of the neuroscientific research is now a bit dated, Damasio's everyday-life descriptions are compelling and still accurate. See also E. Thompson, *Mind in Life: Biology, Phenomenology, and the Sciences of Mind* (Cambridge, MA: Belknap Press of Harvard University Press, 2007); and F. J. Varela, E. Thompson, and E. Rosch, *The Embodied Mind: Cognitive Science and Human Experience* (Cambridge, MA: MIT Press, 1991).

22 In his essay "The Depth of a Smile," my Catalan family-physician colleague Francesc Borrell-Carrió described what he called a "smile of accommodation." See F. Borrell-Carrió, "The Depth of a Smile," *Medical Encounter* 15(2) (2000): 13–14.

23 A. M. Glenberg et al., "Grounding Language in Bodily States: The Case for Emotion," in *Grounding Cognition: The Role of Perception and Action in Memory, Language, and Thinking*, eds. D. Pecher and R. A. Zwaan (Cambridge: Cambridge University Press, 2005).

24 L. Nielsen and A. Kasvniak, "Awareness of Subtle Emotional Feelings: A Comparison of Long-term Meditators and Nonmeditators," *Emotion* 6(3) (2006): 392–405.

25 P. M. Niedenthal, "Embodying Emotion," *Science* 316(5827) (2007): 1002–5.

26 G. Kramer, *Insight Dialogue: The Interpersonal Path to Freedom* (Boulder, CO: Shambhala Publications, 2007).

27 D. L. Cooperrider and D. Whitney, *Appreciative Inquiry: A Positive Revolution in Change* (San Francisco: Berrett-Koehler, 2005).

28 R. M. Epstein, "Making the Ineffable Visible," *Families Systems and Health* 33(3) (2015): 280–82; and J. Zlatev et al., *The Shared Mind: Perspectives on Intersubjectivity* (Amsterdam and Philadelphia: John Benjamins, 2008).

29 J. L. Coulehan, "Tenderness and Steadiness: Emotions in Medical Practice," *Literature and Medicine* 14(2) (1995): 222–36.

30 See G. C. Spivak, L. E. Lyons, and C. G. Franklin, "'On the Cusp of the Personal and the Impersonal': An Interview with Gayatri Chakravorty Spivak," *Biography* 27(1) (2004): 203–21; and R. M. Epstein, "Realizing Engel's Biopsychosocial Vision: Resilience, Compassion, and Quality of Care," *International Journal of Psychiatry in Medicine* 47(4) (2014): 275–87.

31 M. K. Kearney et al., "Self-Care of Physicians Caring for Patients at the End of Life: 'Being Connected . . . a Key to My Survival,'" *JAMA* 301(11) (2009): 1155–64.

32 Coulehan, "Tenderness and Steadiness."

33 W. Steig, *Doctor De Soto* (New York: Square Fish, 2010).

12. IMAGINING A MINDFUL HEALTH CARE SYSTEM

1 See Institute of Medicine, *Crossing the Quality Chasm: A New Health System for the 21st Century* (Washington, DC: National Academies Press, 2001); D. M. Berwick, T. W. Nolan, and J. Whittington, "The Triple Aim: Care, Health, and Cost," *Health Affairs* 27(3) (2008): 759–69; and T. Bodenheimer and C. Sinsky, "From Triple to Quadruple Aim: Care of the Patient Requires Care of the Provider," *Annals of Family Medicine* 12(6) (2014): 573–76.

2 For three of the most influential documents, see Institute of Medicine, *Crossing the Quality Chasm*: Berwick, Nolan, and Whittington, "Triple Aim"; and Bodenheimer and Sinsky, "From Triple to Quadruple Aim."

3 See K. E. Weick and K. H. Roberts, "Collective Mind in Organizations—Heedful Interrelating on Flight Decks," *Administrative Science Quarterly* 38(3) (1993): 357–81. The actual reference to this particular story is G. I. Rochlin, T. R. La Porte, and K. H. Roberts, "The Self-Designing High-Reliability Organization: Aircraft Carrier Flight Operations at Sea," *Naval War College Review* 51(3) (1998): 97.

4 L. T. Kohn, J. M. Corrigan, and M. S. Donaldson, *To Err Is Human: Building a Safer Health System* (Washington, DC: National Academy Press, 2000).

5 K. E. Weick and T. Putnam, "Organizing for Mindfulness: Eastern Wisdom and Western Knowledge," *Journal of Management Inquiry* 15(3) (2006): 275–87; and K. E. Weick and K. M. Sutcliffe, "Mindfulness and the Quality of Organizational Attention," *Organization Science* 17(4) (2006): 514–24.

6 See Weick and Sutcliffe, "Mindfulness and the Quality of Organizational Attention"; D. J. Good et al., "Contemplating Mindfulness at Work: An Integrative Review," *Journal of Management* (2015): 1–29; T. J. Vogus and K. M. Sutcliffe, "Organizational Resilience: Towards a Theory and Research Agenda" (paper presented at the 2007 IEEE International Conference on Systems, Man and Cybernetics, Montreal, Quebec, 2007); T. J. Vogus and K. M. Sutcliffe, "Organizational Mindfulness and Mindful Organizing: A Reconciliation and Path Forward," *Academy of Management Learning & Education* 11(4) (2012): 722–35; and K. M. Weick and K. M. Sutcliffe, *Managing the Unexpected: Assuring High Performance in an Age of Complexity* (San Francisco: Jossey-Bass, 2001).

7 T. J. Vogus and K. M. Sutcliffe, "The Safety Organizing Scale: Development and Validation of a Behavioral Measure of Safety Culture in Hospital Nursing Units," *Medical Care* 45(1) (2007): 46–54.

8 This approach was made famous by Toyota in the 1990s. See the *Harvard Business Review* article at https://hbr.org/1999/09/decoding-the-dna-of-the-toyota-production-system.

9 In case you're worried, the patient went immediately to the emergency room and recovered well.

10 T. J. Vogus and K. M. Sutcliffe, "The Impact of Safety Organizing, Trusted Leadership, and Care Pathways on Reported Medication Errors in Hospital Nursing Units," *Medical Care* 45(10) (2007): 997–1002; and Vogus and Sutcliffe, "Safety Organizing Scale."

11 Here are some references to Suchman's work, which clearly has relevance to other enterprises, not just health care: A. L. Suchman, "Organizations as Machines, Organizations as Conversations: Two Core Metaphors and Their Consequences," *Medical Care* 49 (2011): S43–S48; K. Marvel et al., "Relationship-Centered Administration: Transferring Effective Communication Skills from the Exam Room to the Conference Room," *Journal of Healthcare Management/American College of Healthcare Executives* 48(2) (2002): 112–23, and discussion, 23–24; A. L. Suchman, "The Influence of Health Care Organizations on Well-Being," *Western Journal of Medicine* 174(1) (2001): 43; A. L. Suchman, D. J. Sluyter, and P. R. Williamson, *Leading Change in Healthcare: Transforming Organizations Using Complexity, Positive Psychology, and Relationship-Centered Care* (Abingdon, UK: Radcliffe Publishing, 2011); and A. L. Suchman and P. R. Williamson, "Principles and Practices of Relationship-Centered Meetings" (Rochester, NY: Relationship Centered Health Care, 2006.)

12 D. L. Cooperrider and D. Whitney, *Appreciative Inquiry: A Positive Revolution in Change* (San Francisco: Berrett-Koehler, 2005).

13 Other—secular—health systems are increasingly appointing "chief empathy officers," directors of "the patient experience," and others in similar roles to focus on enhancing trust, communication, and healing relationships.

14 See K. B. Schwartz, "A Patient's Story," *Boston Globe Magazine*, 1995, 16; and Schwartz Center for Compassionate Healthcare, http://www.theschwartz center.org, for further information about the foundation.

15 B. A. Lown and C. F. Manning, "The Schwartz Center Rounds: Evaluation of an Interdisciplinary Approach to Enhancing Patient-Centered Communication, Teamwork, and Provider Support," *Academic Medicine* 85(6) (2010): 1073–81.

16 Monash University, the largest medical school in Australia, and the University of Rochester, where I work, have been the pioneers. At Rochester, we offer five required mindful practice workshops in the third year of medical school. We also offer four- and five-day workshops for practicing physicians and educators who wish to develop their skills further. For information about Rochester's mindful practice programs, see www.mindfulpractice.urmc .edu. Here are a few sample websites for programs that promote well-being in clinicians: http://www.medicine.virginia.edu/administration/faculty/fac ulty-dev/copy_of_home-page; http://www.ohsu.edu/xd/education/schools /school-of-medicine/gme-cme/gme/resident-fellow-wellness-program /index.cfm; http://www.tfme.org/regional-conferences/physician-well-be ing-conference; and http://www.mayo.edu/research/centers-programs/phy sician-well-being-program/overview. For general information about mindfulness and medical education, see P. L. Dobkin and T. A. Hutchinson, "Teaching Mindfulness in Medical School: Where Are We Now and Where Are We Going," *Medical Education* 47(8) (2013): 768–79.

APPENDIX: ATTENTION PRACTICE

1 R. M. Epstein, "Mindful Practice," *JAMA* 282(9) (1999): 833–39.
2 One accessible guide to different meditation practices for psychotherapists is S. M. Pollak, T. Pedulla, and R. D. Siegel, *Sitting Together: Essential Skills for Mindfulness-Based Psychotherapy* (New York: Guilford Press, 2014). For audio files from our programs, please go to https://www.urmc.rochester .edu/family-medicine/mindful-practice/curricula-materials/audios.aspx. On the Web, guided meditations can be found at http://www.mindfulness-solu tion.com/DownloadMeditations.html and https://www.tarabrach.com/guid ed-meditations. For shorter meditations, try http://marc.ucla.edu/body.cfm ?id=22. A popular app for beginning meditators is "Headspace"—compelling and entertaining.

Reference List

Abramson, L. Y., M. E. Seligman, and J. D. Teasdale. "Learned Helplessness in Humans: Critique and Reformulation." *Journal of Abnormal Psychology* 87(1) (1978): 49–74.

Adams, J. R., G. Elwyn, F. Legare, and D. L. Frosch. "Communicating with Physicians about Medical Decisions: A Reluctance to Disagree." *Archives of Internal Medicine* 172(15) (2012): 1184–86.

Allen, T. J., J. W. Sherman, F. R. Conrey, and S. J. Stroessner. "Stereotype Strength and Attentional Bias: Preference for Confirming versus Disconfirming Information Depends on Processing Capacity." *Journal of Experimental Social Psychology* 45(5) (2009): 1081–87.

Aristotle. *The Nicomachean Ethics,* trans. David Ross. Revised with an introduction and notes by Lesley Brown. New York: Oxford University Press, 2009.

Austin, J. H. *Zen and the Brain: Toward an Understanding of Meditation and Consciousness.* Cambridge, MA: MIT Press, 1998.

Baars, B. J., T. Z. Ramsoy, and S. Laureys. "Brain, Conscious Experience and the Observing Self." *Trends in Neurosciences* 26(12) (2003): 671–75.

Babbott, S., L. B. Manwell, R. Brown, E. Montague, E. Williams, M. Schwartz, E. Hess, and M. Linzer. "Electronic Medical Records and Physician Stress in Primary Care: Results from the Memo Study." *Journal of the American Medical Informatics Association* 21(e1) (2014): e100–e106.

Bachman, K. H., and D. K. Freeborn. "HMO Physicians' Use of Referrals." *Social Science & Medicine* 48(4) (1999): 547–57.

Back, A. L., S. M. Bauer-Wu, C. H. Rushton, and J. Halifax. "Compassionate Silence in the Patient-Clinician Encounter: A Contemplative Approach." *Journal of Palliative Medicine* 12(12) (2009): 1113–17.

Back, A. L., C. H. Rushton, A. W. Kaszniak, and J. S. Halifax. "'Why Are We Doing This?': Clinician Helplessness in the Face of Suffering." *Journal of Palliative Medicine* 18(1) (2015): 26–30.

Baker, D. B., R. Day, and E. Salas. "Teamwork as an Essential Component of High-Reliability Organizations." *Health Services Research* 41(4, pt. 2) (2006): 1576–98.

Balint, M. *The Doctor, His Patient, and the Illness.* New York: International Universities Press, 1957.

Banaji, M., and A. Greenwald. *Blindspot: Hidden Biases of Good People*. New York: Delacorte Press, 2013.

Barks, C. *The Essential Rumi*. London: Castle Books, 1997.

Baron, R. J. "An Introduction to Medical Phenomenology: I Can't Hear You While I'm Listening." *Annals of Internal Medicine* 103(4) (1985): 606–11.

Bartels, J. "Eloquent Silences: A Musical and Lexical Analysis of Conversation between Oncologists and Their Patients." *Patient Education & Counseling* (forthcoming, 2016).

Bartz, J. A., J. Zaki, N. Bolger, E. Hollander, N. N. Ludwig, A. Kolevzon, and K. N. Ochsner. "Oxytocin Selectively Improves Empathic Accuracy." *Psychological Science* 21(10) (2010): 1426–28.

Bassler, D., J. W. Busse, P. J. Karanicolas, and G. H. Guyatt. "Evidence-Based Medicine Targets the Individual Patient. Part 2: Guides and Tools for Individual Decision-Making." *ACP Journal Club* 149(1) (2008): 2.

Batchelor, S. *Buddhism without Beliefs: A Contemporary Guide to Awakening*. New York: Riverhead Books, 1997.

Batson, D. C. "These Things Called Empathy: Eight Related but Distinct Phenomena." In *The Social Neuroscience of Empathy*, edited by J. Decety and W. Ickes, chap. 1, 3–15. Denver, CO: Bradford, 2009.

Baumgarten, E. "Curiosity as a Moral Virtue." *International Journal of Applied Philosophy* 15(2) (2001): 23–42.

Beach, M. C., D. Roter, P. T. Korthuis, R. M. Epstein, V. Sharp, N. Ratanawongsa, J. Cohn, et al. "A Multicenter Study of Physician Mindfulness and Health Care Quality." *Annals of Family Medicine* 11(5) (2013): 421–28.

Beckman, H. B., K. M. Markakis, A. L. Suchman, and R. M. Frankel. "The Doctor-Patient Relationship and Malpractice: Lessons from Plaintiff Depositions." *Archives of Internal Medicine* 154(12) (1994): 1365–70.

Beckman, H. B., M. Wendland, C. Mooney, M. S. Krasner, T. E. Quill, A. L. Suchman, and R. M. Epstein. "The Impact of a Program in Mindful Communication Primary Care Physicians." *Academic Medicine* 87(6) (2012): 1–5.

Bereiter, C., and M. Scardamalia. *Surpassing Ourselves: An Inquiry into the Nature and Implications of Expertise*. Chicago: Open Court Publishing, 1993.

Berger, J. E., and R. L. Boyle Jr. "How to Avoid the High Costs of Physician Turnover." *Medical Group Management Journal* 39(6) (1991): 80–82.

Berlyne, D. E. "Novelty and Curiosity as Determinants of Exploratory Behaviour." *British Journal of Psychiatry* 41(1–2) (1950): 68–80.

Berry, D. L., D. J. Wilkie, C. R. J. Thomas, and P. Fortner. "Clinicians Communicating with Patients Experiencing Cancer Pain." *Cancer Investigation* 21(3) (2003): 374–81.

Berwick, D. M., T. W. Nolan, and J. Whittington. "The Triple Aim: Care, Health, and Cost." *Health Affairs* 27(3) (2008): 759–69.

Bilek, E., M. Ruf, A. Schafer, C. Akdeniz, V. D. Calhoun, C. Schmahl, C. Demanuele, et al. "Information Flow between Interacting Human Brains: Identification, Validation, and Relationship to Social Expertise." *Proceedings of the National Academy of Sciences* 112(16) (2015): 5207–12.

Bodenheimer, T., and C. Sinsky. "From Triple to Quadruple Aim: Care of the

Patient Requires Care of the Provider." *Annals of Family Medicine* 12(6) (2014): 573–76.

Borrell-Carrió, F. "The Depth of a Smile." *Medical Encounter* 15(2) (2000): 13–14.

Borrell-Carrió, F., and R. M. Epstein. "Preventing Errors in Clinical Practice: A Call for Self-Awareness." *Annals of Family Medicine* 2(4) (2004): 310–16.

Brewer, A., and K. Garrison. "The Posterior Cingulate Cortex as a Plausible Mechanistic Target of Meditation: Findings from Neuroimaging." *Annals of the New York Academy of Sciences* 1307(1) (2014): 19–27.

Brown, K. W., and R. M. Ryan. "The Benefits of Being Present: Mindfulness and Its Role in Psychological Well-Being." *Journal of Personality and Social Psychology* 84(4) (2003): 822–48.

Buber, M. *I and Thou*. New York: Scribner, 1970.

Buchbinder, S. B., M. Wilson, C. F. Melick, and N. R. Powe. "Estimates of Costs of Primary Care Physician Turnover." *American Journal of Managed Care* 5(11) (1999): 1431–38.

Burgess, D. J. "Are Providers More Likely to Contribute to Healthcare Disparities under High Levels of Cognitive Load? How Features of the Healthcare Setting May Lead to Biases in Medical Decision Making." *Medical Decision Making* 30(2) (2010): 246–57.

Burgess, D. J., S. S. Fu, and M. van Ryn. "Why Do Providers Contribute to Disparities and What Can Be Done about It?" *Journal of General Internal Medicine* 19(11) (2004): 1154–59.

Candib, L. M. "Working with Suffering." *Patient Education & Counseling* 48(1) (2002): 43–50.

Caspi, A., and B. W. Roberts. "Personality Development across the Life Course: The Argument for Change and Continuity." *Psychological Inquiry* 12(2) (2001): 49–66.

Cassell, E. J. "Diagnosing Suffering: A Perspective." *Annals of Internal Medicine* 131(7) (1999): 531–34.

———. "The Nature of Suffering and the Goals of Medicine." *New England Journal of Medicine* 306(11) (1982): 639–45.

———. "The Phenomenon of Suffering and Its Relationship to Pain." In *Handbook of Phenomenology and Medicine*, edited by S. K. Toombs, 371–90. Dordrecht, Netherlands: Kluwer Academic Publishers, 2001.

Catlin, A., C. Armigo, D. Volat, E. Vale, M. A. Hadley, W. Gong, R. Bassir, and K. Anderson. "Conscientious Objection: A Potential Neonatal Nursing Response to Care Orders That Cause Suffering at the End of Life? Study of a Concept." *Neonatal Network—Journal of Neonatal Nursing* 27(2) (2008): 101–8.

Chabris, C., and D. Simons. *The Invisible Gorilla: How Our Intuitions Deceive Us*. New York: Crown, 2011.

Charlin, B., H. P. Boshuizen, E. J. Custers, and P. J. Feltovich. "Scripts and Clinical Reasoning." *Medical Education* 41(12) (2007): 1178–84.

Charon, R. "Narrative Medicine: Form, Function, and Ethics." *Annals of Internal Medicine* 134(1) (2001): 83–87.

———. *Narrative Medicine: Honoring the Stories of Illness*. London: Oxford University Press, 2006.

Chatel-Goldman J., J. L. Schwartz, C. Jutten, and M. Congedo. "Non-Local Mind from the Perspective of Social Cognition." *Frontiers in Human Neuroscience* 7 (2013): 107.

Cheng, Y., C.-Y. Yang, C.-P. Lin, P.-L. Lee, and J. Decety. "The Perception of Pain in Others Suppresses Somatosensory Oscillations: A Magnetoencephalography Study." *NeuroImage* 40(4) (2008): 1833–40.

Chou, C. M., K. Kellom, and J. A. Shea. "Attitudes and Habits of Highly Humanistic Physicians." *Academic Medicine* 89(9) (2014): 1252–58.

Cicchetti, D., and F. A. Rogosch. "Gene × Environment Interaction and Resilience: Effects of Child Maltreatment and Serotonin, Corticotropin Releasing Hormone, Dopamine, and Oxytocin Genes." *Development and Psychopathology* 24(2) (2012): 411–27.

Clance, P. R. *The Impostor Phenomenon: When Success Makes You Feel Like a Fake*. New York: Bantam Books, 1986.

Connelly, J. "Being in the Present Moment: Developing the Capacity for Mindfulness in Medicine." *Academic Medicine* 74(4) (1999): 420–24.

Connelly, J. E. "The Guest House (Commentary)." *Academic Medicine* 83(6) (2008): 588–89.

———. "Narrative Possibilities: Using Mindfulness in Clinical Practice." *Perspectives in Biology and Medicine* 48(1) (2005): 84–94.

Cooperrider, D. L., and D. Whitney. *Appreciative Inquiry: A Positive Revolution in Change*. San Francisco: Berrett-Koehler, 2005.

Corbetta, M., and G. L. Shulman. "Control of Goal-Directed and Stimulus-Driven Attention in the Brain." *Nature Reviews Neuroscience* 3(3) (2002): 201–15.

Costa, P. T., and R. R. McCrae. "NEO PI-R: Professional Manual, Revised Neo Personality Inventory (NEO PI-R), and Neo Five-Factor Inventory (NEO-FFI)." Odessa, FL: Psychological Assessment Resources, 1992.

Coulehan, J. "Compassionate Solidarity: Suffering, Poetry, and Medicine." *Perspectives in Biology and Medicine* 52(4) (2009): 585–603.

Coulehan, J. L. "Tenderness and Steadiness: Emotions in Medical Practice." *Literature and Medicine* 14(2) (1995): 222–36.

Croskerry, P. "Clinical Cognition and Diagnostic Error: Applications of a Dual Process Model of Reasoning." *Advances in Health Sciences Education* 14(1) (2009): 27–35.

———. "Context Is Everything or How Could I Have Been That Stupid?" *Healthcare Quarterly* 12 (2009): e171–e76.

———. "From Mindless to Mindful Practice—Cognitive Bias and Clinical Decision Making." *New England Journal of Medicine* 368(26) (2013): 2445–48.

———. "The Importance of Cognitive Errors in Diagnosis and Strategies to Minimize Them." *Academic Medicine* 78(8) (2003): 775–80.

———. "A Universal Model of Diagnostic Reasoning." *Academic Medicine* 84(8) (2009): 1022–28.

Croskerry, P., A. A. Abbass, and A. W. Wu. "How Doctors Feel: Affective Issues in Patients' Safety." *Lancet* 372(9645) (2008): 1205–6.

Croskerry, P., and G. R. Nimmo. "Better Clinical Decision Making and Reducing Diagnostic Error." *Journal of the Royal College of Physicians of Edinburgh* 41(2) (2011): 155–62.

Croskerry, P., and G. Norman. "Overconfidence in Clinical Decision Making." *American Journal of Medicine* 121(5) (2008): S24–S29.

Damasio, A. R. *Descartes' Error: Emotion, Reason, and the Human Brain*. New York: G. P. Putnam's Sons, 1994.

———. *The Feeling of What Happens: Body and Emotion in the Making of Consciousness*. New York: Harcourt Brace, 1999.

Darley, J. M., and C. D. Batson. "'From Jerusalem to Jericho': A Study of Situation and Dispositional Variables in Helping Behavior." *Journal of Personality and Social Psychology* 27(1) (1973): 100–108.

Davidson, R. J. "Anterior Cerebral Asymmetry and the Nature of Emotion." *Brain and Cognition* 20(1) (1992): 125–51.

Davidson, R. J., J. Kabat-Zinn, J. Schumacher, M. Rosenkranz, D. Muller, S. F. Santorelli, F. Urbanowski, et al. "Alterations in Brain and Immune Function Produced by Mindfulness Meditation." *Psychosomatic Medicine* 65(4) (2003): 564–70.

Davidson, R. J., and A. W. Kaszniak. "Conceptual and Methodological Issues in Research on Mindfulness and Meditation." *American Psychologist* 70(7) (2015): 581–92.

Decety, J., and C. Lamm. "Empathy Versus Personal Distress: Recent Evidence from Social Neuroscience." In *The Social Neuroscience of Empathy*, edited by J. Decety and W. Ickes, chap. 15, 199–213. Denver, CO: Bradford, 2009.

Decety, J., C. Y. Yang, and Y. Cheng. "Physicians Down-Regulate Their Pain Empathy Response: An Event-Related Brain Potential Study." *NeuroImage* 50(4) (2010): 1676–82.

Deci, E. L., and R. M. Ryan. *Intrinsic Motivation and Self-Determination in Human Behavior*. New York: Plenum Press, 1985.

De Dreu, C. K. "Oxytocin Modulates Cooperation within and Competition between Groups: An Integrative Review and Research Agenda." *Hormones and Behavior* 61(3) (2012): 419–28.

De Jaegher, H., and E. Di Paolo. "Participatory Sense-Making: An Enactive Approach to Social Cognition." *Phenomenology and the Cognitive Sciences* 6(4) (2007): 485–507.

de Vignemont, F., and T. Singer. "The Empathic Brain: How, When and Why?" *Trends in Cognitive Sciences* 10(10) (2006): 435–41.

Dewey, J. *Experience and Nature*. New York: Dover, 1958.

DeYoung, C. G., D. Cicchetti, F. A. Rogosch, J. R. Gray, M. Eastman, and E. L. Grigorenko. "Sources of Cognitive Exploration: Genetic Variation in the Prefrontal Dopamine System Predicts Openness/Intellect." *Journal of Research in Personality* 45(4) (2011): 364–71.

Dimsdale, J. E. "Reflections on the Impact of Antihypertensive Medications on Mood, Sedation, and Neuropsychologic Functioning." *Archives of Internal Medicine* 152(1) (1992): 35–39.

Dixon, C. A. J., C. N. E. Tompkins, V. L. Allgar, and N. M. J. Wright. "Abusive Behaviour Experienced by Primary Care Receptionists: A Cross-Sectional Survey." *Family Practice* 21(2) (2004): 137–39.

Dobkin, P. L., and T. A. Hutchinson. "Teaching Mindfulness in Medical School:

Where Are We Now and Where Are We Going." *Medical Education* 47(8) (2013): 768–79.

Dovidio, J. F., K. Kawakami, C. Johnson, B. Johnson, and A. Howard. "On the Nature of Prejudice: Automatic and Controlled Processes." *Journal of Experimental Social Psychology* 33(5) (1997): 510–40.

Drew, T., M. L. Vo, and J. M. Wolfe. "The Invisible Gorilla Strikes Again: Sustained Inattentional Blindness in Expert Observers." *Psychological Science* 24(9) (2013): 1848–53.

Dreyfus, H. L. *On the Internet (Thinking in Action)*. New York: Routledge, 2001.

Dyche, L., and R. M. Epstein. "Curiosity and Medical Education." *Medical Education* 45(7) (2011): 663–68.

Dyrbye, L. N., F. S. Massie, A. Eacker, W. Harper, D. Power, S. J. Durning, M. R. Thomas, et al. "Relationship between Burnout and Professional Conduct and Attitudes among US Medical Students." *JAMA* 304(11) (2010): 1173–80.

Dyrbye, L. N., M. R. Thomas, F. S. Massie, D. V. Power, A. Eacker, W. Harper, S. Durning, et al. "Burnout and Suicidal Ideation among US Medical Students." *Annals of Internal Medicine* 149(5) (2008): 334–41.

Dyrbye, L. N., P. Varkey, S. L. Boone, D. V. Satele, J. A. Sloan, and T. D. Shanafelt. "Physician Satisfaction and Burnout at Different Career Stages." *Mayo Clinic Proceedings* 88(12) (2013): 1358–67.

Dyrbye, L. N., C. P. West, D. Satele, S. Boone, L. Tan, J. Sloan, and T. D. Shanafelt. "Burnout among US Medical Students, Residents, and Early Career Physicians Relative to the General US Population." *Academic Medicine* 89(3) (2014): 443–51.

Ebstein, R. P., O. Novick, R. Umansky, B. Priel, Y. Osher, D. Blaine, E. R. Bennett, et al. "Dopamine D4 Receptor (D4DR) Exon III Polymorphism Associated with the Human Personality Trait of Novelty Seeking." *Nature Genetics* 12(1) (1996): 78–80.

Eisenberg, N., and N. D. Eggum. "Empathic Responding: Sympathy and Personal Distress." In *The Social Neuroscience of Empathy*, edited by J. Decety and W. Ickes, chap. 6, 71–83. Denver, CO: Bradford, 2009.

Elliot, A. J., and H. T. Reis. "Attachment and Exploration in Adulthood." *Journal of Personality and Social Psychology* 85(2) (2003): 317–31.

Elwyn, G., A. O'Connor, D. Stacey, R. Volk, A. Edwards, A. Coulter, R. Thomson, et al. "Developing a Quality Criteria Framework for Patient Decision Aids: Online International Delphi Consensus Process." *British Medical Journal* 333(7565) (2006): 417.

Engel, G. L. "The Clinical Application of the Biopsychosocial Model." *American Journal of Psychiatry* 137(5) (1980): 535–44.

———. "From Biomedical to Biopsychosocial: Being Scientific in the Human Domain." *Psychosomatics* 38(6) (1997): 521–28.

———. "The Need for a New Medical Model: A Challenge for Biomedicine." *Science* 196(4286) (1977): 129–36.

———. "What If Music Students Were Taught to Play Their Instruments as Medical Students Are Taught to Interview?" *Pharos of Alpha Omega Alpha Honor Medical Society* (1982), 4512–13.

Engen, H. G., and T. Singer. "Compassion-Based Emotion Regulation Up-

Regulates Experienced Positive Affect and Associated Neural Networks." *Social Cognitive and Affective Neuroscience* 10(9) (2015): 1291–301.

Epstein, M. *Thoughts without a Thinker: Psychotherapy from a Buddhist Perspective*. New York: Basic Books, 1995.

Epstein, R. M. "Making the Ineffable Visible." *Families Systems and Health* 33(3) (2015): 280–82.

———. "Mindful Practice." *JAMA* 282(9) (1999): 833–39.

———. "Physician Know Thy Family: Looking at One's Family-of-Origin as a Method of Physician Self-Awareness." *Medical Encounter* 8(1) (1991): 9.

———. "Realizing Engel's Biopsychosocial Vision: Resilience, Compassion, and Quality of Care." *International Journal of Psychiatry in Medicine* 47(4) (2014): 275–87.

———. "Whole Mind and Shared Mind in Clinical Decision-Making." *Patient Education & Counseling* 90(2) (2013): 200–206.

Epstein, R. M., B. S. Alper, and T. E. Quill. "Communicating Evidence for Participatory Decision Making." *JAMA* 291(19) (2004): 2359–66.

Epstein, R. M., and A. L. Back. "Responding to Suffering." *JAMA* 314(24) (2015): 2623–24.

Epstein, R. M., M. Christie, R. Frankel, S. Rousseau, C. Shields, and A. L. Suchman. "Understanding Fear of Contagion among Physicians Who Care for HIV Patients." *Family Medicine* 25(4) (1993): 264–68.

Epstein, R. M., E. F. Dannefer, A. C. Nofziger, J. T. Hansen, S. H. Schultz, N. Jospe, L. W. Connard, et al. "Comprehensive Assessment of Professional Competence: The Rochester Experiment." *Teaching and Learning in Medicine* 16(2) (2004): 186–96.

Epstein, R. M., P. Franks, K. Fiscella, C. G. Shields, S. C. Meldrum, R. L. Kravitz, and P. R. Duberstein. "Measuring Patient-Centered Communication in Patient-Physician Consultations: Theoretical and Practical Issues." *Social Science & Medicine* 61(7) (2005): 1516–28.

Epstein, R. M., and R. E. Gramling. "What Is Shared in Shared Decision Making? Complex Decisions When the Evidence Is Unclear." *Medical Care Research and Review* 70(1S) (2012): 94–112.

Epstein, R. M., T. Hadee, J. Carroll, S. C. Meldrum, J. Lardner, and C. G. Shields. "'Could This Be Something Serious?' Reassurance, Uncertainty, and Empathy in Response to Patients' Expressions of Worry." *Journal of General Internal Medicine* 22(12) (2007): 1731–39.

Epstein, R. M., and E. M. Hundert. "Defining and Assessing Professional Competence." *JAMA* 287(2) (2002): 226–35.

Epstein, R. M., D. S. Morse, R. M. Frankel, L. Frarey, K. Anderson, and H. B. Beckman. "Awkward Moments in Patient-Physician Communication about HIV Risk." *Annals of Internal Medicine* 128(6) (1998): 435–42.

Epstein, R. M., T. E. Quill, and I. R. McWhinney. "Somatization Reconsidered: Incorporating the Patient's Experience of Illness." *Archives of Internal Medicine* 159(3) (1999): 215–22.

Epstein, R. M., C. G. Shields, S. C. Meldrum, K. Fiscella, J. Carroll, P. A. Carney, and P. R. Duberstein. "Physicians' Responses to Patients' Medically Unexplained Symptoms." *Psychosomatic Medicine* 68(2) (2006): 269–76.

Reference List

Epstein, R. M., D. J. Siegel, and J. Silberman. "Self-Monitoring in Clinical Practice: A Challenge for Medical Educators." *Journal of Continuing Education in the Health Professions* 28(1) (2008): 5–13.

Epstein, R. M., and R. L. Street Jr. "Shared Mind: Communication, Decision Making, and Autonomy in Serious Illness." *Annals of Family Medicine* 9(5) (2011): 454–61.

Eraut, M. *Developing Professional Knowledge and Competence.* London: Falmer Press, 1994.

Ericsson, K. A. "An Expert-Performance Perspective of Research on Medical Expertise: The Study of Clinical Performance." *Medical Education* 41(12) (2007): 1124–30.

Fahrenkopf, A. M., T. C. Sectish, L. K. Barger, P. J. Sharek, D. Lewin, V. W. Chiang, S. Edwards, et al. "Rates of Medication Errors among Depressed and Burnt-Out Residents: Prospective Cohort Study." *BMJ* 1(7642) (2008): 488–91.

Farber, S. "Living Every Minute." *Journal of Pain and Symptom Management* 49(4) (2015): 796–800.

Feder, A., E. J. Nestler, and D. S. Charney. "Psychobiology and Molecular Genetics of Resilience." *Nature Reviews Neuroscience* 10(6) (2009): 446–57.

Festinger, L. "Cognitive Dissonance." *Scientific American* 207(4) (1962): 93–107.

Fitzgerald, F. S. "The Crack Up." In *The Crack Up*, edited by E. Wilson. New York: New Directions, 1945.

Fitzgerald, F. T. "Curiosity." *Annals of Internal Medicine* 130(1) (1999): 70–72.

Fonagy, P., G. Gergely, E. Jurist, and M. Target. *Affect Regulation, Mentalization, and the Development of Self.* New York: Other Press, 2002.

Foucault, M. *The Birth of the Clinic: An Archaeology of Medical Perception.* New York: Random House, 1994.

Fox, R. *Experiment Perilous: Physicians and Patients Facing the Unknown.* Glencoe, IL: Free Press, 1959.

Frank, A. W. "Can We Research Suffering?" *Qualitative Health Research* 11(3) (2001): 353–62.

Friedberg, M. W., P. G. Chen, K. R. Van Busum, F. M. Aunon, C. Pham, J. P. Caloyeras, S. Mattke, et al. "Factors Affecting Physician Professional Satisfaction and Their Implications for Patient Care, Health Systems, and Health Policy." 2013. http://www.rand.org/content/dam/rand/pubs/research_reports/RR400/RR439/RAND_RR439.pdf.

Fronsdal, G. "Not-Knowing." http://www.insightmeditationcenter.org/books-articles/articles/not-knowing.

Fry, J. P. "Interactive Relationship between Inquisitiveness and Student Control of Instruction." *Journal of Educational Psychology* 68(5) (1972): 459–65.

Fukushima, H., Y. Terasawa, and S. Umeda. "Association between Interoception and Empathy: Evidence from Heartbeat-Evoked Brain Potential." *International Journal of Psychophysiology* 79(2) (2011): 259–65.

Gabbard, G. O. "The Role of Compulsiveness in the Normal Physician." *JAMA* 254(20) (1985): 2926–29.

Gabel, S. "Demoralization: A Precursor to Physician Burnout?" *American Family Physician* 86(9) (2012): 861–62.

Reference List

Gallagher, T. H., A. D. Waterman, A. G. Ebers, V. J. Fraser, and W. Levinson. "Patients' and Physicians' Attitudes regarding the Disclosure of Medical Errors." *JAMA* 289(8) (2003): 1001–7.

Germer, C. K. *The Mindful Path to Self-Compassion: Freeing Yourself from Destructive Thoughts and Emotions.* New York: Guilford Press, 2009.

Gerrity, M. S., R. F. DeVellis, and J. A. Earp. "Physicians' Reactions to Uncertainty in Patient Care. A New Measure and New Insights." *Medical Care* 28(8) (1990): 724–36.

Gillett, G. "Clinical Medicine and the Quest for Certainty." *Social Science & Medicine* 58(4) (2004): 727–38.

Glenberg, A. M., D. Havas, R. Becker, and M. Rinck. "Grounding Language in Bodily States: The Case for Emotion." In *Grounding Cognition: The Role of Perception and Action in Memory, Language, and Thinking*, edited by Diane Pecher and Rolf A. Zwaan. Cambridge: Cambridge University Press, 2005.

Glouberman, S., and B. Zimmerman. "Complicated and Complex Systems: What Would Successful Reform of Medicare Look Like?" In *Romanow Papers: Changing Health Care in Canada*, edited by Pierre-Gerlier Forest, Gregory P. Marchildon, and Tom McIntosh. Toronto: University of Toronto Press, 2002.

Goldberg, P. *The Intuitive Edge: Understanding and Developing Intuition.* Los Angeles: J. P. Tarcher, 1983.

Goldberg, S. B., A. C. Del Re, W. T. Hoyt, and J. M. Davis. "The Secret Ingredient in Mindfulness Interventions? A Case for Practice Quality over Quantity." *Journal of Counseling Psychology* 61(3) (2014): 491–97.

Good, D. J., C. J. Lyddy, T. M. Glomb, J. E. Bono, K. W. Brown, M. K. Duffy, R. A. Baer, et al. "Contemplating Mindfulness at Work: An Integrative Review." *Journal of Management* 42(1) (2015): 1–29.

Gordon, G. H., S. K. Joos, and J. Byrne. "Physician Expressions of Uncertainty during Patient Encounters." *Patient Education & Counseling* 40(1) (2000): 59–65.

Gorenstein, D. "How Doctors Die: Showing Others the Way." *New York Times*, November 19, 2013. http://www.nytimes.com/2013/11/20/your-money/how-doctors-die.html?_r=2.

Gottlieb, J., P.-Y. Oudeyer, M. Lopes, and A. Baranes. "Information-Seeking, Curiosity, and Attention: Computational and Neural Mechanisms." *Trends in Cognitive Sciences* 17(11) (2013): 585–93.

Granek, L. "When Doctors Grieve." *New York Times*, May 27, 2012.

Granek, L., P. Mazzotta, R. Tozer, and M. K. Krzyzanowska. "What Do Oncologists Want?" *Supportive Care in Cancer* 20(10) (2012): 2627–32.

Granek, L., R. Tozer, P. Mazzotta, A. Ramjaun, and M. Krzyzanowska. "Nature and Impact of Grief over Patient Loss on Oncologists' Personal and Professional Lives." *Archives of Internal Medicine* 172(12) (2012): 964–66.

Green, A. R., D. R. Carney, D. J. Pallin, L. H. Ngo, K. L. Raymond, L. I. Iezzoni, and M. R. Banaji. "Implicit Bias among Physicians and Its Prediction of Thrombolysis Decisions for Black and White Patients." *Journal of General Internal Medicine* 22(9) (2007): 1231–38.

Greenberg, J., and N. Meiran. "Is Mindfulness Meditation Associated with 'Feeling Less'?" *Mindfulness* 5(5) (2014): 471–76.

Greenberg, J., K. Reiner, and N. Meiran. "'Mind the Trap': Mindfulness Practice Reduces Cognitive Rigidity." *PLoS ONE* 7(5) (2012): e36206.

Greene, J. *Moral Tribes: Emotion, Reason, and the Gap between Us and Them.* New York: Penguin Press, 2013.

Greenwald, A. G., D. E. McGhee, and J. L. K. Schwartz. "Measuring Individual Differences in Implicit Cognition: The Implicit Association Test." *Journal of Personality and Social Psychology* 74(6) (1998): 1464–80.

Groopman, J. E. *How Doctors Think.* New York: Houghton Mifflin, 2007.

Grossman, P. "On Measuring Mindfulness in Psychosomatic and Psychological Research." *Journal of Psychosomatic Research* 64(4) (2008): 405–8.

Guyatt, G., V. Montori, P. J. Devereaux, H. Schunemann, and M. Bhandari. "Patients at the Center: In Our Practice, and in Our Use of Language." *ACP Journal Club* 140(1) (2004): A11–A12.

Haas, J. S., E. F. Cook, A. L. Puopolo, H. R. Burstin, P. D. Cleary, and T. A. Brennan. "Is the Professional Satisfaction of General Internists Associated with Patient Satisfaction?" *Journal of General Internal Medicine* 15(2) (2000): 122–28.

Hafenbrack, A. C., Z. Kinias, and S. G. Barsade. "Debiasing the Mind through Meditation Mindfulness and the Sunk-Cost Bias." *Psychological Science* 25(2) (2014): 369–76.

Haidet, P. "Jazz and the 'Art' of Medicine: Improvisation in the Medical Encounter." *Annals of Family Medicine* 5(2) (2007): 164–69.

Halifax, J. *Being with Dying.* Boulder, CO: Shambhala Publications, 2008.

———. "A Heuristic Model of Enactive Compassion." *Current Opinion in Supportive and Palliative Care* 6(2) (2012): 228–35.

Hall, W. J., M. V. Chapman, K. M. Lee, Y. M. Merino, T. W. Thomas, B. K. Payne, E. Eng, et al. "Implicit Racial/Ethnic Bias among Health Care Professionals and Its Influence on Health Care Outcomes: A Systematic Review." *American Journal of Public Health* 105(12) (2015): e60–e76.

Halpern, J. *From Detached Concern to Empathy: Humanizing Medical Practice.* Oxford: Oxford University Press, 2001.

———. "What Is Clinical Empathy?" *Journal of General Internal Medicine* 18(8) (2003): 670–74.

Harlow, J. M. "Recovery after Severe Injury to the Head." *History of Psychiatry* (1993): 274–81. (Originally published 1868 in the *Bulletin of the Massachusetts Medical Society*).

Harper, R. *On Presence: Variations and Reflections.* Philadelphia: Trinity Press International, 1991.

Harris, S. *Waking Up: A Guide to Spirituality without Religion.* New York: Simon & Schuster, 2015.

Hatano, G., and K. Inagaki. "Child Development and Education in Japan." In *Two Courses of Expertise*, edited by H. Stevenson, H. Azuma, and K. Hakuta, 262–72. New York: Freeman, 1986.

Haynes, R. B., D. L. Sackett, D. W. Taylor, E. S. Gibson, and A. L. Johnson. "Increased Absenteeism from Work after Detection and Labeling of

Hypertensive Patients." *New England Journal of Medicine* 299(14) (1978): 741–44.

Hebb, D. *The Organization of Behavior.* New York: Wiley, 1949.

Hill, R. G. Jr., L. M. Sears, and S. W. Melanson. "4,000 Clicks: A Productivity Analysis of Electronic Medical Records in a Community Hospital ED." *American Journal of Emergency Medicine* 31(11) (2013): 1591–94.

Ho, B., and E. Liu. "Does Sorry Work? The Impact of Apology Laws on Medical Malpractice." *Journal of Risk and Uncertainty* 43(2) (2011): 141–67.

Hojat, M., D. Z. Louis, F. W. Markham, R. Wender, C. Rabinowitz, and J. S. Gonnella. "Physicians' Empathy and Clinical Outcomes for Diabetic Patients." *Academic Medicine* 86(3) (2011): 359–64.

Hojat, M., M. J. Vergare, K. Maxwell, G. Brainard, S. K. Herrine, G. A. Isenberg, J. Veloski, et al. "The Devil Is in the Third Year: A Longitudinal Study of Erosion of Empathy in Medical School." *Academic Medicine* 84(9) (2009): 1182–91.

Hölzel, B. K., S. W. Lazar, T. Gard, Z. Schuman-Olivier, D. R. Vago, and U. Ott. "How Does Mindfulness Meditation Work? Proposing Mechanisms of Action from a Conceptual and Neural Perspective." *Perspectives on Psychological Science* 6(6) (2011): 537–59.

Horowitz, C. R., A. L. Suchman, W. T. Branch Jr., and R. M. Frankel. "What Do Doctors Find Meaningful about Their Work?" *Annals of Internal Medicine* 138(9) (2003): 772–75.

Howard, S. K., D. M. Gaba, K. J. Fish, G. Yang, and F. H. Sarnquist. "Anesthesia Crisis Resource Management Training: Teaching Anesthesiologists to Handle Critical Incidents." *Aviation, Space, and Environmental Medicine* 63(9) (1992): 763–70.

Institute of Medicine. *Crossing the Quality Chasm: A New Health System for the 21st Century.* Washington, DC: National Academies Press, 2001.

Ismail-Beigi, F., E. Moghissi, M. Tiktin, I. B. Hirsch, S. E. Inzucchi, and S. Genuth. "Individualizing Glycemic Targets in Type 2 Diabetes Mellitus: Implications of Recent Clinical Trials." *Annals of Internal Medicine* 154(8) (2011): 554–59.

James, W. "Brute and Human Intellect." In *William James: Writings 1878–1899.* New York: Library of America, 1992.

———. *Pragmatism.* Cambridge, MA: Harvard University Press, 1975.

———. *The Principles of Psychology.* Cambridge, MA: Harvard University Press, 1981.

———. *The Varieties of Religious Experience: A Study in Human Nature.* New York: W. W. Norton, 1902; repr., 1961.

———. *William James: The Essential Writings.* Albany: State University of New York Press, 1986.

James, W. M. "Brute and Human Intellect." *Journal of Speculative Philosophy* 12(3) (1878): 236–76.

Jha, A. P., A. B. Morrison, J. Dainer-Best, S. Parker, N. Rostrup, and E. A. Stanley. "Minds 'at Attention': Mindfulness Training Curbs Attentional Lapses in Military Cohorts." *PLoS ONE* 10(2) (2015): e0116889.

Jha, A. P., E. A. Stanley, A. Kiyonaga, L. Wong, and L. Gelfand. "Examining the

Protective Effects of Mindfulness Training on Working Memory Capacity and Affective Experience." *Emotion* 10(1) (2010): 54–64.

Johansen, M. L., K. A. Holtedahl, A. S. Davidsen, and C. E. Rudebeck. "'I Deal with the Small Things': The Doctor-Patient Relationship and Professional Identity in GPs' Stories of Cancer Care." *Health* 16(6) (2012): 569–84.

Johnson, C. G., J. C. Levenkron, A. L. Suchman, and R. Manchester. "Does Physician Uncertainty Affect Patient Satisfaction?" *Journal of General Internal Medicine* 3(2) (1988): 144–49.

Johnson, D. C., N. J. Thom, E. A. Stanley, L. Haase, A. N. Simmons, P.-A. B. Shih, W. K. Thompson, et al. "Modifying Resilience Mechanisms in At-Risk Individuals: A Controlled Study of Mindfulness Training in Marines Preparing for Deployment." *American Journal of Psychiatry* 171(8) (2014): 844–53.

Kabat-Zinn, J. *Full Catastrophe Living: Using the Wisdom of Your Body and Mind to Face Stress, Pain, and Illness.* New York: Bantam Dell, 1990.

———. *Wherever You Go, There You Are: Mindfulness Meditation in Everyday Life.* New York: Hyperion, 1994.

Kahneman, D. "A Perspective on Judgment and Choice: Mapping Bounded Rationality." *American Psychologist* 58(9) (2003): 697–720.

———. *Thinking, Fast and Slow.* New York: Farrar, Straus and Giroux, 2013.

Kahneman, D., and G. Klein. "Conditions for Intuitive Expertise: A Failure to Disagree." *American Psychologist* 64(6) (2009): 515–26.

Kandel, E. R. "A New Intellectual Framework for Psychiatry." *American Journal of Psychiatry* 155(4) (1998): 457–69.

Kang, Y., J. R. Gray, and J. F. Dovidio. "The Nondiscriminating Heart: Loving-kindness Meditation Training Decreases Implicit Intergroup Bias." *Journal of Experimental Psychology: General* 143(3) (2014): 1306.

Kang, Y., J. Gruber, and J. R. Gray. "Mindfulness and De-automatization." *Emotion Review* 5(2) (2013): 192–201.

Kaptchuk, T. J. *The Web That Has No Weaver: Understanding Chinese Medicine.* New York: Congdon & Weed, 1983.

Karan, S. B., J. S. Berger, and M. Wajda. "Confessions of Physicians: What Systemic Reporting Does Not Uncover." *Journal of Graduate Medical Education* 7(4) (2015): 528–30.

Kashdan, T. B., A. Afram, K. W. Brown, M. Birnbeck, and M. Drvoshanov. "Curiosity Enhances the Role of Mindfulness in Reducing Defensive Responses to Existential Threat." *Personality and Individual Differences* 50(8) (2011): 1227–32.

Kassirer, J. P. "Our Stubborn Quest for Diagnostic Certainty. A Cause of Excessive Testing." *New England Journal of Medicine* 320(22) (1989): 1489–91.

Kaszniak, A. W. "Meditation, Mindfulness, Cognition, and Emotion: Implications for Community-Based Older Adult Programs." In *Enhancing Cognitive Fitness in Adults*, edited by Paula E. Hartman-Stein and Asenath LaRue, chap. 5, 85–104. New York: Springer, 2011.

Katon, W., M. Sullivan, and E. Walker. "Medical Symptoms without Identified Pathology: Relationship to Psychiatric Disorders, Childhood and Adult Trauma, and Personality Traits." *Annals of Internal Medicine* 134(9, pt. 2) (2001): 917–25.

Reference List

Kearney, M. K., R. B. Weininger, M. L. Vachon, R. L. Harrison, and B. M. Mount. "Self-Care of Physicians Caring for Patients at the End of Life: 'Being Connected . . . a Key to My Survival.'" *JAMA* 301(11) (2009): 1155–64.

Kelley, J. M., G. Kraft-Todd, L. Schapira, J. Kossowsky, and H. Riess. "The Influence of the Patient-Clinician Relationship on Healthcare Outcomes: A Systematic Review and Meta-analysis of Randomized Controlled Trials." *PLoS ONE* 9(4) (2014).

Kemper, K. J., and M. Khirallah. "Acute Effects of Online Mind-Body Skills Training on Resilience, Mindfulness, and Empathy." *Journal of Evidence-Based Complementary & Alternative Medicine* 20(4) (2015): 247–53.

Kidd, C., and B. Y. Hayden. "The Psychology and Neuroscience of Curiosity." *Neuron* 88(3) (2015): 449–60.

Kleinman, A. M. *The Illness Narratives: Suffering, Healing, and the Human Condition*. New York: Basic Books, 1988.

Klimecki, O. M., S. Leiberg, M. Ricard, and T. Singer. "Differential Pattern of Functional Brain Plasticity after Compassion and Empathy Training." *Social Cognitive and Affective Neuroscience* 9(6) (2014): 873–79.

Klitzman, R. *When Doctors Become Patients*. New York: Oxford University Press, 2008.

Kohn, L. T., J. M. Corrigan, and M. S. Donaldson. *To Err Is Human: Building a Safer Health System*. Washington, DC: National Academy Press, 2000.

Komesaroff, P. "The Many Faces of the Clinic: A Levinasian View." In *Handbook of Phenomenology and Medicine*, edited by S. K. Toombs, 317–30. Dordrecht, Netherlands: Kluwer Academic Publishers, 2001.

Kramer, G. *Insight Dialogue: The Interpersonal Path to Freedom*. Boulder, CO: Shambhala Publications, 2007.

Krasner, M. S., R. M. Epstein, H. Beckman, A. L. Suchman, B. Chapman, C. J. Mooney, and T. E. Quill. "Association of an Educational Program in Mindful Communication with Burnout, Empathy, and Attitudes among Primary Care Physicians." *JAMA* 302(12) (2009): 1284–93.

Kübler-Ross, E., S. Wessler, and L. V. Avioli. "On Death and Dying." *JAMA* 221 (1972): 174–79.

Kushnir, T., D. Greenberg, N. Madjar, I. Hadari, Y. Yermiahu, and Y. G. Bachner. "Is Burnout Associated with Referral Rates among Primary Care Physicians in Community Clinics?" *Family Practice* 31(1) (2014): 44–50.

Lamm, C., C. D. Batson, and J. Decety. "The Neural Substrate of Human Empathy: Effects of Perspective-Taking and Cognitive Appraisal." *Journal of Cognitive Neuroscience* 19(1) (2007): 42–58.

Lamm, C., A. N. Meltzoff, and J. Decety. "How Do We Empathize with Someone Who Is Not Like Us? A Functional Magnetic Resonance Imaging Study." *Journal of Cognitive Neuroscience* 22(2) (2010): 362–76.

Langer, E. J. *Mindfulness*. Reading, MA: Addison-Wesley, 1989.

———. *The Power of Mindful Learning*. Reading, MA: Perseus Books, 1997.

Larson, E. B., and X. Yao. "Clinical Empathy as Emotional Labor in the Patient-Physician Relationship." *JAMA* 293(9) (2005): 1100–106.

Leary, M. R., E. B. Tate, C. E. Adams, A. Batts Allen, and J. Hancock. "Self-Compassion and Reactions to Unpleasant Self-Relevant Events: The Implications of Treating Oneself Kindly." *Journal of Personality and Social Psychology* 92(5) (2007): 887.

Lee, T. H. "The Word That Shall Not Be Spoken." *New England Journal of Medicine* 369(19) (2013): 1777–79.

Leff, J., G. Williams, M. A. Huckvale, M. Arbuthnot, and A. P. Leff. "Computer-Assisted Therapy for Medication-Resistant Auditory Hallucinations: Proof-of-Concept Study." *British Journal of Psychiatry* 202(6) (2013): 428–33.

Legassie, J., E. M. Zibrowski, and M. A. Goldszmidt. "Measuring Resident Well-Being: Impostorism and Burnout Syndrome in Residency." *Journal of General Internal Medicine* 23(7) (2008): 1090–94.

Leonard, N. H., and M. Harvey. "Curiosity, Mindfulness and Learning Style in the Acquisition of Knowledge by Individuals/Organisations. *International Journal of Learning and Intellectual Capital* 4(3) (2007): 294–314.

Lesser, M. *Know Yourself, Forget Yourself: Five Truths to Transform Your Work, Relationships, and Everyday Life*. Novato, CA: New World Library, 2013.

Leung, A. S. O., R. M. Epstein, and C. A. Moulton. "The Competent Mind: Beyond Cognition." In *The Question of Competence: Reconsidering Medical Education in the Twenty-First Century*, edited by B. D. Hodges and L. Lingard, chap. 7, 155–76. Ithaca and London: Cornell University Press, 2012.

Levinson, W., R. Gorawara-Bhat, and J. Lamb. "A Study of Patient Clues and Physician Responses in Primary Care and Surgical Settings." *JAMA* 284(8) (2000): 1021–27.

Levitin, D. J. *The Organized Mind: Thinking Straight in the Age of Information Overload*. New York: Dutton Adult, 2014.

Levy, D. M., J. O. Wobbrock, A. W. Kaszniak, and M. Ostergren. "The Effects of Mindfulness Meditation Training on Multitasking in a High-Stress Information Environment." In *Proceedings of Graphics Interface 2012*, 45–52. Toronto: Canadian Information Processing Society, 2012.

Lichtenstein, R. L. "Review Article: The Job Satisfaction and Retention of Physicians in Organized Settings: A Literature Review." *Medical Care Research and Review* 41(3) (1984): 139–79.

Lindblom, C. E. "The Science of 'Muddling Through.'" *Public Administration Review* 19(2) (1959): 79–88.

Linzer, M., M. R. Visser, F. J. Oort, E. M. Smets, J. E. McMurray, and H. C. de Haes. "Predicting and Preventing Physician Burnout: Results from the United States and the Netherlands." *American Journal of Medicine* 111(2) (2001): 170–75.

Lown, B. A., and C. F. Manning. "The Schwartz Center Rounds: Evaluation of an Interdisciplinary Approach to Enhancing Patient-Centered Communication, Teamwork, and Provider Support." *Academic Medicine* 85(6) (2010): 1073–81.

Lown, B. A., J. Rosen, and J. Marttila. "An Agenda for Improving Compassionate Care: A Survey Shows About Half of Patients Say Such Care Is Missing." *Health Affairs* 30(9) (2011): 1772–78.

Lueke, A., and B. Gibson. "Mindfulness Meditation Reduces Implicit Age and

Race Bias: The Role of Reduced Automaticity of Responding." *Social Psychological and Personality Science* (2014): 1–8.

Lutz, A., L. L. Greischar, D. M. Perlman, and R. J. Davidson. "Bold Signal in Insula Is Differentially Related to Cardiac Function during Compassion Meditation in Experts vs. Novices." *NeuroImage* 47(3) (2009): 1038–46.

Macdonald, J. S., and N. Lavie. "Visual Perceptual Load Induces Inattentional Deafness." *Attention, Perception, and Psychophysics* 73(6) (2011): 1780–89.

Maguire, E. A., K. Woollett, and H. J. Spiers. "London Taxi Drivers and Bus Drivers: A Structural MRI and Neuropsychological Analysis." *Hippocampus* 16(12) (2006): 1091–101.

Mancini, A. D., and G. A. Bonanno. "Predictors and Parameters of Resilience to Loss: Toward an Individual Differences Model." *Journal of Personality* 77(6) (2009): 1805–32.

Marvel, K., A. Bailey, C. Pfaffly, W. Gunn, and H. Beckman. "Relationship-Centered Administration: Transferring Effective Communication Skills from the Exam Room to the Conference Room." *Journal of Healthcare Management/American College of Healthcare Executives* 48(2) (2002): 112–23; discussion, 23–24.

Marvel, M. K., R. M. Epstein, K. Flowers, and H. B. Beckman. "Soliciting the Patient's Agenda: Have We Improved?" *JAMA* 281(3) (1999): 283–87.

Maslach, C. "Job Burnout." *Current Directions in Psychological Science* 12(5) (2003): 189–92.

Maslach, C., S. Jackson, and M. Leiter. "Maslach Burnout Inventory: Third Edition." In *Evaluating Stress: A Book of Resources*, edited by C. P. Zalaquett and R. J. Wood, 191–218. Lanham, MD: Scarecrow Press, 1998.

Maslach, C., W. B. Schaufeli, and M. P. Leiter. "Job Burnout." *Annual Review of Psychology* (2001): 52397–422.

Maue, K. *Water in the Lake: Real Events for the Imagination.* New York: Harper & Row, 1979.

McCrae, R. R., and P. T. Costa Jr. "Personality Trait Structure as a Human Universal." *American Psychologist* 52(5) (1997): 509–16.

McCrae, R. R., P. T. Costa Jr., F. Ostendorf, A. Angleitner, M. Hrebickova, M. D. Avia, J. Sanz, et al. "Nature over Nurture: Temperament, Personality, and Life Span Development." *Journal of Personality and Social Psychology* 78(1) (2000): 173–86.

McDaniel, S. H., H. B. Beckman, D. S. Morse, J. Silberman, D. B. Seaburn, and R. M. Epstein. "'Enough about Me, Let's Get Back to You': Physician Self-Disclosure during Primary Care Encounters." *Annals of Internal Medicine* 149(11) (2008): 835–37.

McDaniel, S. H., T. L. Campbell, and D. B. Seaburn. *Family-Oriented Primary Care: A Manual for Medical Providers.* New York: Springer-Verlag, 1990.

McDaniel, S. H., and J. Landau-Stanton. "Family-of-Origin Work and Family Therapy Skills Training: Both-And." *Family Process* 30(4) (1991): 459–71.

McHugh, M. D., A. Kutney-Lee, J. P. Cimiotti, D. M. Sloane, and L. H. Aiken. "Nurses' Widespread Job Dissatisfaction, Burnout, and Frustration with Health Benefits Signal Problems for Patient Care." *Health Affairs* 30(2) (2011): 202–10.

McMurray, J. E., M. Linzer, T. R. Konrad, J. Douglas, R. Shugerman, and K. Nelson. "The Work Lives of Women Physicians: Results from the Physician Work Life Study. The SGIM Career Satisfaction Study Group." *Journal of General Internal Medicine* 15(6) (2000): 372–80.

McWhinney, I. R. "Fifty Years On: The Legacy of Michael Balint." *British Journal of General Practice* 49 (1999): 418–19.

McWhinney, I. R., R. M. Epstein, and T. R. Freeman. "Rethinking Somatization." *Advances in Mind-Body Medicine* 17(4) (2001): 232–39.

Mengel, M. "Physician Ineffectiveness due to Family-of-Origin Issues." *Family Systems Medicine* 5(2) (1987): 176–90.

Michaelson, L. K., A. B. Knight, and D. Flink. *Team-Based Learning: A Transformative Use of Small Groups.* New York: Praeger, 2002.

Milgram, S. "Behavioral Study of Obedience." *Journal of Abnormal Psychology* (1963): 67371–78.

Mohanty, A., T. Egner, J. M. Monti, and M. M. Mesulam. "Search for a Threatening Target Triggers Limbic Guidance of Spatial Attention." *Journal of Neuroscience* 29(34) (2009): 10563–72.

Mohanty, A., and T. J. Sussman. "Top-Down Modulation of Attention by Emotion." *Frontiers in Human Neuroscience* 7 (2013): 102.

Montgomery, K. "Thinking about Thinking: Implications for Patient Safety." *Healthcare Quarterly* (Toronto, Canada) 12 (2008): e191–e194.

Montori, V. M., and G. H. Guyatt. "Progress in Evidence-Based Medicine." *JAMA* 300(15) (2008): 1814–16.

Morse, D. S., E. A. Edwardsen, and H. S. Gordon. "Missed Opportunities for Interval Empathy in Lung Cancer Communication." *Archives of Internal Medicine* 168(17) (2008): 1853–58.

Moulton, C. A., and R. M. Epstein. "Self-Monitoring in Surgical Practice: Slowing Down When You Should." In *Surgical Education: Theorising an Emerging Domain*, edited by H. Fry and R. Kneebone, chap. 10, 169–82. New York: Springer, 2011.

Moulton, C. A., G. Regehr, M. Mylopoulos, and H. M. MacRae. "Slowing Down When You Should: A New Model of Expert Judgment." *Academic Medicine RIME: Proceedings of the Forty-Sixth Annual Conference* 82(10) (2007): S109–S116.

Mujica-Parodi, L. R., H. H. Strey, B. Frederick, R. Savoy, D. Cox, Y. Botanov, D. Tolkunov, et al. "Chemosensory Cues to Conspecific Emotional Stress Activate Amygdala in Humans." *PLoS ONE* 4(7) (2009): e6415.

Mulligan, N. W. "The Role of Attention during Encoding in Implicit and Explicit Memory." *Journal of Experimental Psychology: Learning, Memory, & Cognition* 21(1) (1998): 27–47.

Murray, K. "How Doctors Die—It's Not Like the Rest of Us, but It Should Be." *Zócalo Public Square*, November 30, 2011, 1775–77.

Naef, R. "Bearing Witness: A Moral Way of Engaging in the Nurse-Person Relationship." *Nursing Philosophy* 7(3) (2006): 146–56.

Nedrow, A., N. A. Steckler, and J. Hardman. "Physician Resilience and Burnout: Can You Make the Switch?" *Family Practice Management* 20(1) (2013): 25–30.

Neff, K. D., and C. K. Germer. "A Pilot Study and Randomized Controlled Trial of the Mindful Self-Compassion Program." *Journal of Clinical Psychology* 69(1) (2013): 28–44.

Neff, K. D., Y.-P. Hsieh, and K. Dejitterat. "Self-Compassion, Achievement Goals, and Coping with Academic Failure." *Self and Identity* 4(3) (2005): 263–87.

Niedenthal, P. M. "Embodying Emotion." *Science* 316(5827) (2007): 1002–5.

Niemiec, C. P., K. W. Brown, T. B. Kashdan, P. J. Cozzolino, W. E. Breen, C. Levesque-Bristol, and R. M. Ryan. "Being Present in the Face of Existential Threat: The Role of Trait Mindfulness in Reducing Defensive Responses to Mortality Salience." *Journal of Personality and Social Psychology* 99(2) (2010): 344–65.

Nin, A. *The Diary of Anaïs Nin, 1939–1944*. New York: Harcourt, Brace & World, 1969.

Norman, G., M. Young, and L. Brooks. "Non-analytical Models of Clinical Reasoning: The Role of Experience." *Medical Education* 41(12) (2007): 1140–45.

Novack, D. H., R. M. Epstein, and R. H. Paulsen. "Toward Creating Physician-Healers: Fostering Medical Students' Self-Awareness, Personal Growth, and Well-Being." *Academic Medicine* 74(5) (1999): 516–20.

Novack, D. H., C. Kaplan, R. M. Epstein, W. Clark, A. L. Suchman, M. O'Brien, E. Najberg, et al. "Personal Awareness and Professional Growth: A Proposed Curriculum." *Medical Encounter* 13(3) (1997): 2–7.

Novack, D. H., A. L. Suchman, W. Clark, R. M. Epstein, E. Najberg, and C. Kaplan. "Calibrating the Physician. Personal Awareness and Effective Patient Care." *JAMA* 278(6) (1997): 502–9.

Ofri, D. "The Epidemic of Disillusioned Doctors." *Time*, 2013. Published electronically July 2, 2013. http://ideas.time.com/2013/07/02/the-epidemic -of-disillusioned-doctors.

Ogden, J., K. Fuks, M. Gardner, S. Johnson, M. McLean, P. Martin, and R. Shah. "Doctors' Expressions of Uncertainty and Patient Confidence." *Patient Education & Counseling* 48(2) (2002): 171–76.

Olson, K., K. J. Kemper, and J. D. Mahan. "What Factors Promote Resilience and Protect against Burnout in First-Year Pediatric and Medicine-Pediatric Residents?" *Journal of Evidence-Based Complementary & Alternative Medicine* 20(3) (2015): 192–98.

Oord, T. J. *Defining Love: A Philosophical, Scientific, and Theological Engagement*. Ada, MI: Brazos Press, 2010.

O'Rourke, M. "Doctors Tell All—and It's Bad." *Atlantic*, November 2014. http:// www.theatlantic.com/magazine/archive/2014/11/doctors-tell-all-and-its- bad/380785.

Pembroke, N. "Human Dimension in Medical Care: Insights from Buber and Marcel." *Southern Medical Journal* 103(12) (2010): 1210–13.

Pence, G. E. "Can Compassion Be Taught?" *Journal of Medical Ethics* 9(4) (1983): 189–91.

"Physician Wellness Services and Cejka Search. 2011 Physician Stress and Burnout Survey." 2011. http://www.cejkasearch.com/wp-content/uploads/physician -stress-burnout-survey.pdf.

Physicians Foundation. "A Survey of America's Physicians: Practice Patterns and

Perspectives, an Examination of the Professional Morale, Practice Patterns, Career Plans, and Healthcare Perspectives of Today's Physicians, Aggregated by Age, Gender, Primary Care/Specialists, and Practice Owners/ Employees." 2012. http://www.physiciansfoundation.org/uploads/default /Physicians_Foundation_2012_Biennial_Survey.pdf.

Polanyi, M. "Knowing and Being, the Logic of Tacit Inference." In *Knowing and Being: Essays by Michael Polanyi*, edited by M. Grene, chaps. 9 and 10, 123– 58. Chicago: University of Chicago Press, 1969.

———. *Personal Knowledge: Towards a Post-critical Philosophy*. Chicago: University of Chicago Press, 1974.

———. *The Tacit Dimension*. Gloucester, MA: Peter Smith, 1983.

Pollak, S. M., T. Pedulla, and R. D. Siegel. *Sitting Together: Essential Skills for Mindfulness-Based Psychotherapy*. New York: Guilford Press, 2014.

Pololi, L. H., E. Krupat, J. T. Civian, A. S. Ash, and R. T. Brennan. "Why Are a Quarter of Faculty Considering Leaving Academic Medicine? A Study of Their Perceptions of Institutional Culture and Intentions to Leave at 26 Representative US Medical Schools." *Academic Medicine* 87(7) (2012): 859–69.

Price, M. C. "Intuitive Decisions on the Fringes of Consciousness: Are They Conscious and Does It Matter?" *Judgment and Decision Making* 3(1) (2008): 28–41.

Prose, N. "Paying Attention." *JAMA* 283(21) (2000): 2763.

Quill, T. E., and H. Brody. "Physician Recommendations and Patient Autonomy: Finding a Balance between Physician Power and Patient Choice." *Annals of Internal Medicine* 125(9) (1996): 763–69.

Quill, T. E., and P. R. Williamson. "Healthy Approaches to Physician Stress." *Archives of Internal Medicine* 150(9) (1990): 1857–61.

Reniers, R. L., B. A. Vollm, R. Elliott, and R. Corcoran. "Empathy, ToM, and Self- Other Differentiation: An fMRI Study of Internal States." *Social Neuroscience* 9(1) (2014): 50–62.

Reps, P., and N. Senzaki. *Zen Flesh, Zen Bones: A Collection of Zen and Pre-Zen Writings*. Clarendon, VT: Tuttle Publishing, 1998.

Reyna, V. F. "A Theory of Medical Decision Making and Health: Fuzzy Trace Theory." *Medical Decision Making* 28(6) (2008): 850–65.

Reyna, V. F., and F. J. Lloyd. "Physician Decision Making and Cardiac Risk: Effects of Knowledge, Risk Perception, Risk Tolerance, and Fuzzy Processing." *Journal of Experimental Psychology: Applied* 12(3) (2006): 179.

Riva, G., J. A. Waterworth, E. L. Waterworth, and F. Mantovani. "From Intention to Action: The Role of Presence." *New Ideas in Psychology* 29(1) (2011): 24–37.

Rochlin, G. I., T. R. La Porte, and K. H. Roberts. "The Self-Designing High- Reliability Organization: Aircraft Carrier Flight Operations at Sea." *Naval War College Review* 51(3) (1998): 97.

Rodenbach, R. A., K. E. Rodenbach, M. A. Tejani, and R. M. Epstein. "Relationships between Personal Attitudes about Death and Communication with Terminally Ill Patients: How Oncology Clinicians Grapple with Mortality." *Patient Education & Counseling* 99(3) (2015): 356–63.

Roman, B., and J. Kay. "Fostering Curiosity: Using the Educator-Learner Relationship to Promote a Facilitative Learning Environment." *Psychiatry: Interpersonal and Biological Processes* 70(3) (2007): 205–8.

Rushton, C. H., A. W. Kaszniak, and J. S. Halifax. "Addressing Moral Distress: Application of a Framework to Palliative Care Practice." *Journal of Palliative Medicine* 16(9) (2013): 1080–88.

———. "A Framework for Understanding Moral Distress among Palliative Care Clinicians." *Journal of Palliative Medicine* 16(9) (2013): 1074–79.

Russ, A. L., A. J. Zillich, M. S. McManus, B. N. Doebbeling, and J. J. Saleem. "Prescribers' Interactions with Medication Alerts at the Point of Prescribing: A Multi-method, In Situ Investigation of the Human-Computer Interaction." *International Journal of Medical Informatics* 81(4) (2012): 232–43.

Russo, S. J., J. W. Murrough, M.-H. Han, D. S. Charney, and E. J. Nestler. "Neurobiology of Resilience." *Nature Neuroscience* 15(11) (2012): 1475–84.

Sabin, J., B. A. Nosek, A. Greenwald, and F. P. Rivara. "Physicians' Implicit and Explicit Attitudes about Race by MD Race, Ethnicity, and Gender." *Journal of Health Care for the Poor and Underserved* 20(3) (2009): 896–913.

Sabin, J. A., F. P. Rivara, and A. G. Greenwald. "Physician Implicit Attitudes and Stereotypes about Race and Quality of Medical Care." *Medical Care* 46(7) (2008): 678–85.

Sackett, D. L., R. B. Haynes, G. H. Guyatt, and P. Tugwell. *Clinical Epidemiology: A Basic Science for Clinical Medicine*. 2nd ed. Boston: Little Brown, 1991.

Saitta, N., and S. D. Hodge. "Efficacy of a Physician's Words of Empathy: An Overview of State Apology Laws." *Journal of the American Osteopathic Association* 112(5) (2012): 302–6.

———. "Physician Apologies." *Practical Lawyer*, December 2011, 35–43.

———. "Is It Unrealistic to Expect a Doctor to Apologize for an Unforeseen Medical Complication?—a Primer on Apologies Laws." *Pennsylvania Bar Association Quarterly*, July 2011, 93–110.

Salmon P. "Patients Who Present Physical Symptoms in the Absence of Physical Pathology: A Challenge to Existing Models of Doctor-Patient Interaction." *Patient Education & Counseling* 39(1) (2000): 105–13.

Salmon P., L. Wissow, J. Carroll, A. Ring, G. M. Humphris, J. C. Davies, and C. F. Dowrick. "Doctors' Responses to Patients with Medically Unexplained Symptoms Who Seek Emotional Support: Criticism or Confrontation?" *General Hospital Psychiatry* 29(5) (2007): 454–60.

Salvucci, D. D., N. A. Taatgen, and J. P. Borst. "Toward a Unified Theory of the Multitasking Continuum: From Concurrent Performance to Task Switching, Interruption, and Resumption." *Proceedings of ACM CHI 2009 Conference on Human Factors in Computing Systems—Understanding UI 2* (2009), 1819–28.

Salzberg, S. *Lovingkindness: The Revolutionary Art of Happiness*. Boston: Shambhala, 1997.

Schattner, A. "My Most Informative Error." *JAMA Internal Medicine* 175(5) (2015): 681.

Scheingold, L. "Balint Work in England: Lessons for American Family Medicine." *Journal of Family Practice* 26(3) (1988): 315–20.

Schon, D. A. *Educating the Reflective Practitioner.* San Francisco: Jossey-Bass, 1987.

———. *The Reflective Practitioner.* New York: Basic Books, 1983.

Schroeder, D. A., E. Stephens, D. Colgan, M. Hunsinger, D. Rubin, and M. S. Christopher. "A Brief Mindfulness-Based Intervention for Primary Care Physicians: A Pilot Randomized Controlled Trial." *American Journal of Lifestyle Medicine* (2016): 1–9.

Schulman, K. A., J. A. Berlin, W. Harless, J. F. Kerner, S. Sistrunk, B. J. Gersh, R. Dube, et al. "The Effect of Race and Sex on Physicians' Recommendations for Cardiac Catheterization." *New England Journal of Medicine* 340(8) (1999): 618–26.

Schwartz, K. B. "A Patient's Story." *Boston Globe Magazine,* 1995, 16.

Schwartz Center for Compassionate Healthcare. http://www.theschwartzcenter.org.

Scott, S. D., L. E. Hirschinger, K. R. Cox, M. McCoig, J. Brandt, and L. W. Hall. "The Natural History of Recovery for the Healthcare Provider 'Second Victim' after Adverse Patient Events." *Quality and Safety in Health Care* 18(5) (2009): 325–30.

Seaburn, D. B., D. Morse, S. H. McDaniel, H. Beckman, J. Silberman, and R. M. Epstein. "Physician Responses to Ambiguous Patient Symptoms." *Journal of General Internal Medicine* 20(6) (2005): 525–30.

Shanafelt, T. D., O. Hasan, L. N. Dyrbye, C. Sinsky, D. Satele, J. Sloan, and C. P. West. "Changes in Burnout and Satisfaction with Work-Life Balance in Physicians and the General US Working Population between 2011 and 2014." *Mayo Clinic Proceedings* 90(12) (2015): 1600–13.

Shanafelt, T. D., C. P. West, J. A. Sloan, P. J. Novotny, G. A. Poland, R. Menaker, T. A. Rummans, et al. "Career Fit and Burnout among Academic Faculty." *Archives of Internal Medicine* 169(10) (2009): 990–95.

Shapiro, J. "Walking a Mile in Their Patients' Shoes: Empathy and Othering in Medical Students' Education." *Philosophy, Ethics, and Humanities in Medicine* 3(1) (2008): 1.

Shapiro, S. L., and G. E. Schwartz. "Mindfulness in Medical Education: Fostering the Health of Physicians and Medical Practice." *Integrative Medicine* 1(3) (1998): 93–94.

Shapiro, S. L., G. E. Schwartz, and G. Bonner. "Effects of Mindfulness-Based Stress Reduction on Medical and Premedical Students." *Journal of Behavioral Medicine* 21(6) (1998): 581–99.

Shatz, C. J. "The Developing Brain." *Scientific American* 267(3) (1992): 60–67.

Shaughnessy, A. F., D. C. Slawson, and L. Becker. "Clinical Jazz: Harmonizing Clinical Experience and Evidence-Based Medicine." *Journal of Family Practice* 47(6) (1998): 425–28.

Shavers, V. L., and M. L. Brown. "Racial and Ethnic Disparities in the Receipt of Cancer Treatment." *Journal of the National Cancer Institute* 94(5) (2002): 334–57.

Shayne, M., and T. E. Quill. "Oncologists Responding to Grief." *Archives of Internal Medicine* 172(12) (2012): 966–67.

Reference List

Sherman, J. W., F. R. Conrey, and C. J. Groom. "Encoding Flexibility Revisited: Evidence for Enhanced Encoding of Stereotype-Inconsistent Information under Cognitive Load." *Social Cognition* 22(2) (2004): 214–32.

Sherwin, S. *No Longer Patient: Feminist Ethics & Health Care*. Philadelphia: Temple University Press, 1992.

Shields, C. G., M. A. Finley, C. M. Elias, C. J. Coker, J. J. Griggs, K. Fiscella, and R. M. Epstein. "Pain Assessment: The Roles of Physician Certainty and Curiosity." *Health Communication* 28(7) (2013): 740–46.

Simon, G. E., and O. Gureje. "Stability of Somatization Disorder and Somatization Symptoms among Primary Care Patients." *Archives of General Psychiatry* 56(1) (1999): 90–95.

Singer, T., and M. Bolz, *Compassion: Bridging Practice and Science*. Munich, Germany: Max Planck Society, 2013.

Singer, T., H. D. Critchley, and K. Preuschoff. "A Common Role of Insula in Feelings, Empathy and Uncertainty." *Trends in Cognitive Sciences* 13(8) (2009): 334–40.

Sirovich, B. E., S. Woloshin, and L. M. Schwartz. "Too Little? Too Much? Primary Care Physicians' Views on US Health Care: A Brief Report." *Archives of Internal Medicine* 171(17) (2011): 1582–85.

Smith, A. K., D. B. White, and R. M. Arnold. "Uncertainty—the Other Side of Prognosis." *New England Journal of Medicine* 368(26) (2013): 2448–50.

Smith, R. C., A. M. Dorsey, J. S. Lyles, and R. M. Frankel. "Teaching Self-Awareness Enhances Learning about Patient-Centered Interviewing." *Academic Medicine* 74(11) (1999): 1242–48.

Smith, R. C., G. Osborn, R. B. Hoppe, J. S. Lyles, L. Van Egeren, R. Henry, D. Sego, et al. "Efficacy of a One-Month Training Block in Psychosocial Medicine for Residents: A Controlled Study." *Journal of General Internal Medicine* 6(6) (1991): 535–43.

Southwick, S. M., and D. S. Charney. *Resilience: The Science of Mastering Life's Greatest Challenges*. Cambridge: Cambridge University Press, 2012.

Spickard, A. Jr., S. G. Gabbe, and J. F. Christensen. "Mid-Career Burnout in Generalist and Specialist Physicians." *JAMA* 288(12) (2002): 1447–50.

Spivak, G. C., L. E. Lyons, and C. G. Franklin. " 'On the Cusp of the Personal and the Impersonal': An Interview with Gayatri Chakravorty Spivak." *Biography* 27(1) (2004): 203–21.

Srivastava, R. "Speaking up—When Doctors Navigate Medical Hierarchy." *New England Journal of Medicine* 368(4) (2013): 302–5.

Stangor, C., and D. McMillan. "Memory for Expectancy-Congruent and Expectancy-Incongruent Information." *Psychological Bulletin* 111(1) (1992): 42–61.

Stanley, E. A. "Mindfulness-Based Mind Fitness Training (MMFT): An Approach for Enhancing Performance and Building Resilience in High Stress Contexts." In *The Wiley Blackwell Handbook of Mindfulness*, edited by A. Ie, C. T. Ngnoumen, and E. J. Langer, 964–85. Hoboken, NJ: Wiley, 2014.

Stanley, E. A., J. M. Schaldach, A. Kiyonaga, and A. P. Jha. "Mindfulness-Based Mind Fitness Training: A Case Study of a High Stress Pre-deployment Military Cohort." *Cognitive and Behavioral Practice* 18(4) (2011): 566–76.

Steig, W. *Doctor De Soto*. New York: Square Fish, 2010.

Stiegler, M. P. "A Piece of My Mind. What I Learned about Adverse Events from Captain Sully: It's Not What You Think." *JAMA* 313(4) (2015): 361–62.

Streng, F. J. *Emptiness: A Study in Religious Meaning*. Nashville, TN: Abingdon Press, 1967.

Suchman, A. L. "The Influence of Health Care Organizations on Well-Being." *Western Journal of Medicine* 174(1) (2001): 43.

——. "Organizations as Machines, Organizations as Conversations: Two Core Metaphors and Their Consequences." *Medical Care* 49 (2011): S43–S48.

Suchman, A. L., K. Markakis, H. B. Beckman, and R. Frankel. "A Model of Empathic Communication in the Medical Interview." *JAMA* 277(8) (1997): 678–82.

Suchman, A. L., and D. A. Matthews. "What Makes the Patient-Doctor Relationship Therapeutic? Exploring the Connexional Dimension of Medical Care." *Annals of Internal Medicine* 108(1) (1988): 125–30.

Suchman, A. L., D. J. Sluyter, and P. R. Williamson. *Leading Change in Healthcare: Transforming Organizations Using Complexity, Positive Psychology, and Relationship-Centered Care*. Abingdon, UK: Radcliffe Publishing, 2011.

Suchman, A. L., and P. R. Williamson. "Principles and Practices of Relationship-Centered Meetings." Rochester, NY: Relationship Centered Health Care, 2006.

Suzuki, S. *Zen Mind, Beginner's Mind*. New York: Weatherhill, 1980.

Swayden, K. J., K. K. Anderson, L. M. Connelly, J. S. Moran, J. K. McMahon, and P. M. Arnold. "Effect of Sitting vs. Standing on Perception of Provider Time at Bedside: A Pilot Study." *Patient Education and Counseling* 86(2) (2012): 166–71.

Sweller, J. "Cognitive Load During Problem Solving: Effects on Learning." *Cognitive Science* 12(2) (1988): 257–85.

Taleb, N. N. *Antifragile: Things That Gain from Disorder*. New York: Random House, 2014.

Tan, C. M. *Search Inside Yourself*. New York: HarperCollins, 2012.

Tang, Y.-Y., B. K. Hölzel, and M. I. Posner. "The Neuroscience of Mindfulness Meditation." *Nature Reviews Neuroscience* 16(4) (2015): 213–25.

Tang, Y.-Y., Y. Ma, Y. Fan, H. Feng, J. Wang, S. Feng, Q. Lu, et al. "Central and Autonomic Nervous System Interaction Is Altered by Short-Term Meditation." *Proceedings of the National Academy of Sciences* 106(22) (2009): 8865–70.

Tang, Y.-Y., Y. Ma, J. Wang, Y. Fan, S. Feng, Q. Lu, Q. Yu, et al. "Short-Term Meditation Training Improves Attention and Self-Regulation." *Proceedings of the National Academy of Sciences* 104(43) (2007): 17152–56.

Thomas, J. T. "Intrapsychic Predictors of Professional Quality of Life: Mindfulness, Empathy, and Emotional Separation." Lexington: University of Kentucky, 2011.

Thompson, E. *Mind in Life: Biology, Phenomenology, and the Sciences of Mind*. Cambridge, MA: Belknap Press of Harvard University Press, 2007.

Thompson, E., and M. Stapleton. "Making Sense of Sense-Making: Reflections on Enactive and Extended Mind Theories." *Topoi* 28(1) (2009): 23–30.

Reference List

Thorne, S. E., M. Kuo, E. A. Armstrong, G. McPherson, S. R. Harris, And T. G. Hislop. "'Being Known': Patients' Perspectives of the Dynamics of Human Connection in Cancer Care." *Psycho-Oncology* 14(10) (2005): 887–98.

Tinetti, M. E., T. R. Fried, and C. M. Boyd. "Designing Health Care for the Most Common Chronic Condition—Multimorbidity." *JAMA* 307(23) (2012): 2493–94.

Todd, K. H., N. Samaroo, and J. R. Hoffman. "Ethnicity as a Risk Factor for Inadequate Emergency Department Analgesia." *JAMA* 269(12) (1993): 1537–39.

Tversky, A., and D. Kahneman. "The Framing of Decisions and the Psychology of Choice." *Science* 211(4481) (1981): 453–58.

Vago, D., and D. Silbersweig. "Self-Awareness, Self-Regulation, and Self-Transcendence (S-Art): A Framework for Understanding the Neurobiological Mechanisms of Mindfulness." *Frontiers in Human Neuroscience* 6(296) (2012): 1–6.

Vaillant, G. E., N. C. Sobowale, and C. McArthur. "Some Psychologic Vulnerabilities of Physicians." *New England Journal of Medicine* 287 (1972): 372–75.

van Ryn, M. "Research on the Provider Contribution to Race/Ethnicity Disparities in Medical Care." *MedCare* 40(1) (2002): I140–I151.

Varcoe, C., B. Pauly, J. Storch, L. Newton, and K. Makaroff. "Nurses' Perceptions of and Responses to Morally Distressing Situations." *Nursing Ethics* 19(4) (2012): 488–500.

Varela, F. J., E. Thompson, and E. Rosch. *The Embodied Mind: Cognitive Science and Human Experience*. Cambridge, MA: MIT Press, 1991.

Ventres, W. B., and R. M. Frankel. "Shared Presence in Physician-Patient Communication: A Graphic Representation." *Families, Systems, & Health* 33(3) (2015): 270–79.

Verghese, A. "Culture Shock—Patient as Icon, Icon as Patient." *New England Journal of Medicine* 359(26) (2008): 2748–51.

Vogus, T. J., and K. M. Sutcliffe. "The Impact of Safety Organizing, Trusted Leadership, and Care Pathways on Reported Medication Errors in Hospital Nursing Units." *Medical Care* 45(10) (2007): 997–1002.

——— . "Organizational Mindfulness and Mindful Organizing: A Reconciliation and Path Forward." *Academy of Management Learning & Education* 11(4) (2012): 722–35.

——— . "Organizational Resilience: Towards a Theory and Research Agenda." Paper presented at the 2007 IEEE International Conference on Systems, Man, and Cybernetics, Montreal, Quebec, 2007.

——— . "The Safety Organizing Scale: Development and Validation of a Behavioral Measure of Safety Culture in Hospital Nursing Units." *Medical Care* 45(1) (2007): 46–54.

Volz, K. G., and G. Gigerenzer. "Cognitive Processes in Decisions under Risk Are Not the Same as in Decisions under Uncertainty." *Frontiers in Decision Neuroscience* 6(105) (2012): 1–6.

Waitzkin, H., and H. Magana. "The Black Box in Somatization: Unexplained Physical Symptoms, Culture, and Narratives of Trauma." *Social Science & Medicine* 45(6) (1997): 811–25.

Waldman, J. D., F. Kelly, S. Aurora, and H. L. Smith. "The Shocking Cost of Turnover in Health Care." *Health Care Management Review* 29(1) (2004): 2–7.

Walker, E. A., W. J. Katon, D. Keegan, G. Gardner, and M. Sullivan. "Predictors of Physician Frustration in the Care of Patients with Rheumatological Complaints." *General Hospital Psychiatry* 19(5) (1997): 315–23.

Wallace, B. A. *The Attention Revolution: Unlocking the Power of the Focused Mind.* Somerville, MA: Wisdom Publications, 2006.

Waterman, A. D., J. Garbutt, E. Hazel, W. C. Dunagan, W. Levinson, V. J. Fraser, and T. H. Gallagher. "The Emotional Impact of Medical Errors on Practicing Physicians in the United States and Canada." *Joint Commission Journal on Quality and Patient Safety* 33(8) (2007): 467–76.

Weick, K. E., and T. Putnam. "Organizing for Mindfulness: Eastern Wisdom and Western Knowledge." *Journal of Management Inquiry* 15(3) (2006): 275–87.

Weick, K. E., and K. H. Roberts. "Collective Mind in Organizations—Heedful Interrelating on Flight Decks." *Administrative Science Quarterly* 38(3) (1993): 357–81.

Weick, K. E., and K. M. Sutcliffe. "Mindfulness and the Quality of Organizational Attention." *Organization Science* 17(4) (2006): 514–24.

———. *Managing the Unexpected: Assuring High Performance in an Age of Complexity.* San Francisco: Jossey-Bass, 2001.

Weiner, S., and A. Schwartz. "Contextual Errors in Medical Decision Making: Overlooked and Understudied." *Academic Medicine: Journal of the Association of American Medical Colleges* 91(5) (2016): 657–62.

Weinstein, N., and R. M. Ryan. "When Helping Helps: Autonomous Motivation for Prosocial Behavior and Its Influence on Well-Being for the Helper and Recipient." *Journal of Personality and Social Psychology* 98(2) (2010): 222–44.

Welie, J. V. "Towards an Ethics of Immediacy. A Defense of a Noncontractual Foundation of the Care Giver–Patient Relationship." *Medicine, Health Care, and Philosophy* 2(1) (1999): 11–19.

Weng, H. Y., A. S. Fox, A. J. Shackman, D. E. Stodola, J. Z. K. Caldwell, M. C. Olson, G. M. Rogers, and R. J. Davidson. "Compassion Training Alters Altruism and Neural Responses to Suffering." *Psychological Science* 24(7) (2013): 1171–80.

West, C. P., M. M. Huschka, P. J. Novotny, J. A. Sloan, J. C. Kolars, and T. M. Habermann. "Association of Perceived Medical Errors with Resident Distress and Empathy: A Prospective Longitudinal Study." *JAMA* 296(9) (2006): 1071–78.

West, C. P., A. D. Tan, T. M. Habermann, J. A. Sloan, and T. D. Shanafelt. "Association of Resident Fatigue and Distress with Perceived Medical Errors." *JAMA* 302(12) (2009): 1294–300.

Williams, E., L. Manwell, T. Konrad, and M. Linzer. "The Relationship of Organizational Culture, Stress, Satisfaction, and Burnout with Physician-Reported Error and Suboptimal Patient Care: Results from the Memo Study." *Health Care Management Review* 32(3) (2007): 203–12.

Williams, E. S., T. R. Konrad, W. E. Scheckler, D. E. Pathman, M. Linzer, J. E. McMurray, M. Gerrity, and M. Schwartz. "Understanding Physicians' Intentions to Withdraw from Practice: The Role of Job Satisfaction, Job Stress, Mental and Physical Health." *Health Care Management Review* 26(1) (2001): 7–19.

Wilson, T. D. "Strangers to Ourselves: Discovering the Adaptive Unconscious." Cambridge, MA: Belknap Press of Harvard University Press, 2002.

Winnicott, D. W. *The Maturational Processes and the Facilitating Environment.* Madison, CT: International Universities Press, 1965.

Woollett, K., and E. A. Maguire. "Acquiring 'the Knowledge' of London's Layout Drives Structural Brain Changes." *Current Biology* 21(24) (2011): 2109–14.

Wu, A. W. "Medical Error: The Second Victim. The Doctor Who Makes the Mistake Needs Help Too." *Western Journal of Medicine* 172(6) (2000): 358.

Wu, G., A. Feder, H. Cohen, J. J. Kim, S. Calderon, D. S. Charney, and A. A. Mathé. "Understanding Resilience." *Frontiers in Behavioral Neuroscience* 7(10) (2013).

Yamada, K. *The Gateless Gate: The Classic Book of Zen Koans.* New York: Simon & Schuster, 2005.

Zlatev, J., T. P. Racine, C. Sinha, and E. Itkonen. "Intersubjectivity: What Makes Us Human?" In *The Shared Mind: Perspectives on Intersubjectivity*, edited by J. Zlatev, T. P. Racine, C. Sinha, and E. Itkonen, chap. 1, 1–14. Amsterdam and Philadelphia: John Benjamins, 2008.

———. *The Shared Mind: Perspectives on Intersubjectivity.* Amsterdam and Philadelphia: John Benjamins, 2008.

Zoppi, K. "Communication about Concerns in Well-Child Visits." Ann Arbor: University of Michigan, 1994.

Index

Index

self-awareness
  biopsychosocial approach to care and, 9
  burnout and lack of, 166
  compassion and, 129
  confessions project for developing, 148
  culture of health care organizations and, 197
  curiosity and, 41, 49
  importance of, 9
  medical education on, 7, 174, 200, 213n19
  mindful practice with, 10
  oncologists and, 152
  reactions of physicians to their mistakes and, 144
self-compassion, 153–54
self-determination, 228n2, 241n25
sensitivity to operations, in organizational mindfulness, 195
Shapiro, Jo, 155
shared mind, 78, 186, 229n15
  decision making using, 93–94, 101, 105
  leap from whole mind to, 187, 190
shared presence, 69, 72, 76, 77, 83–84, 186
Shayne, Michelle, 152
Shields, Cleve, 53
simplification, and organizational mindfulness, 194–95
Singer, Tania, 135, 235n28
Sinsky, Christine, 192
sitting meditation, 8, 82, 120, 184
smiling, and being present, 184
social epigenetics, 49, 165, 221n22
social presence, 77
soldiers, mind-fitness programs for, 174
Southwick, Steve, 164–65
Spivak, G. C., 188
Srivastava, Ranjana, 95
stillness practice, 81–83, 84
stress hormones, 82–83, 165, 174
Suchman, Tony, 11, 68, 197
suffering
  definition of, 113

example of lack of specific diagnosis and continuing, 115–17
experiences in India viewing, 107–8
feeling of helplessness by physicians and, 117–19
inattention to, 112
lack of symptoms and, 111–12
learning to listen to, 123
mindful practice and, 11
pain associated with, 113
persistence of, after cure, 110–11
physicians' acknowledgement of, 119–22
physicians' attending to, 34, 84
physicians' lack of awareness of, 113–15
physicians' presence and sense of intimacy needed for, 72
physicians' understanding of patients', 52, 53, 56
refocusing and reclaiming at end of life and, 122–23
responding to, 107–23
secondary trauma among physicians from, 133
shared decision making and, 88
use of word by physicians, 107, 114
suicidal thoughts, and burnout, 162
suicides
  of patient, psychiatrist's reaction to, 145–46
  of physicians, after medical errors, 146
surgeons
  certainty and, 47
  emotional content of patients' conversations and, 19–20
  example of lack of mindfulness in, 1–3
  example of mindfulness in, 3–5
  expertise and direct supervision of, 179, 180
  focused attention and, 34
  medical errors and suicide by, 146
  peer coaching by, 155
  presence and, 69
  slowing down, 4–5
  time spent on rounds by, 71
  top-down attention and, 24–25

Index